Vitiligo.

Vitiligo causes, remedies, costs and treatment all included.

The complete Vitiligo book.

by

Steve Sunderland

Table of Contents

Table of Contents

Introduction

Vitiligo is often a frustrating condition for patients and dermatologists alike, but things are definitely looking up. Newer treatments are more effective and have fewer side effects. Furthermore, research in the pipeline now is very promising – both in eliminating the causes of vitiligo and forming new approaches to its treatment.

In recent years there has also been a greater focus on the psychological effects of vitiligo on some patients.

As a dermatologist, I encourage patients to receive early treatments, which may stop the progression of the disease and repigment many of their vitiligo patches. I also applaud those who have accepted their remaining spots and just let them be.

I do hope this book is useful for patients and families. Some of the material may appear at first to be "too hard" to read – but this is vitiligo – a lifelong condition with many causes and many approaches to treatment. I find patients who stay abreast of the science behind the disease understand it better and make the best decisions regarding treatment, diet, and sun health. Information is also needed in many communities where few physicians are eager to treat vitiligo.

If I had one wish beyond a cure for vitiligo it would be for it to become as well-known as freckles so that little children wouldn't feel the need to have printed cards explaining vitiligo to pass out to curious strangers.

I hope this book answers all your questions about this disease.

Chapter 1: The Basics

Vitiligo usually begins as a light, smooth spot on the skin. The darker your normal skin, the more noticeable the spot.

If it runs in your family, you'll already know how to pronounce it --- vittle-EYE-go. Otherwise, you've probably never heard of it before.

It's a fairly common condition of the skin – estimates are that 1% to 2% of the world's population has it. It's not contagious or physically painful and it affects women and men equally.

Vitiligo has been known for centuries. Despite its prevalence throughout the world, there are still mysteries surrounding the cause, progression, and its management. Its mysteries have also attracted artists and charlatans throughout history.

The simple story is that the white or pale skin patch is caused by the absence of the pigment melanin from the skin. The cells that manufacture melanin may have died or they may even be dormant.

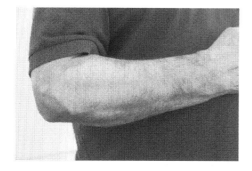

The more complicated story is that vitiligo may also affect the melanin in the eyes, ears, hair, and brain. It may be associated with other conditions. It may progress or it may not and many factors have been identified as its cause. Management is not always simple. And, it may not be vitiligo at all. Presence of white skin patches are caused by several diseases and conditions.

1. Initial Diagnosis of Vitiligo

Diagnosis of vitiligo is often straightforward. Physicians or other health care professionals can make the diagnosis based upon the patient's history and the appearance and distribution of the depigmented areas.

As patches on light skin are sometimes hard to see, a Wood's lamp is often needed to determine the size of the patches and to follow the result of treatment. This lamp gives light in the ultraviolet A range (usually around 365 nanometers) and has a filter to block out almost all visible light. The skin is examined in a dark room, with the examiner having dark-adapted eyes and holding the lamp a few inches from the skin. In normal skin, the skin absorbs the light and no light is reflected back. In vitiligo, there is little or no melanin in the skin so the light is reflected back as a bright blue-white fluorescence.

Unfortunately, this is still where medical care stops for many people with vitiligo. (Or it may stop before the Wood's lamp step.) Many physicians and health insurers still consider vitiligo a cosmetic problem that the patient just has to put up with. This is sad for at least three reasons:

- If caught early, treatment choices and chances of their success are greater.
- Vitiligo can be a sign of an undiagnosed health problem or a harbinger of one to come that should be followed medically.
- Vitiligo presents a serious psychological burden – especially given that it targets very young folks who are at an age when having spotted skin isn't easy to live with.

Books, blogs and articles are full of stories of young people whose initial patches were ignored by their parents, primary care physicians, dermatologists, and school health personnel. Later many of these individuals, having been let down by organized medicine and try homemade treatments on their own.

2. Medical Workup

A full workup of a patient with suspected vitiligo will include medical history, a physical exam, and laboratory tests.

Medical history

At the first visit for this condition, a detailed history of events that preceded the white patch is taken to try to discover a possible trigger. Common triggers include serious sunburn, stress, physical injury or serious illness, and pregnancy. The patient will also be questioned about any symptoms related to autoimmune diseases.

A family history is also taken for vitiligo and any autoimmune disease or prematurely graying hair (Appendix D contains a list of most autoimmune diseases for reference). As discussed in Chapter 4, autoimmune diseases such as thyroid conditions and diabetes are common among families of vitiligo patients. If vitiligo is diagnosed, the patient will be asked routinely about the symptoms of autoimmune diseases.

The effect of vitiligo on the patient

The physician may use conversation and/or a formal questionnaire to elicit how much the vitiligo is bothering the patient and if referral for emotional support is needed. The Dermatology Life Quality Index is a useful tool often used to monitor the impact of the disease; it consists of 10 questions of events during the previous week.

Patients need to be comfortable in order to be honest with their physician and follow the treatment plans. Since the treatments take some time to show promise and may not be effective, they need a good working relationship. Stress is a common trigger of the disease and can also cause flare-ups so it's important for patients to find a physician who doesn't add to the stress.

Physical examination

A total examination of the skin is needed – patients themselves may not be aware of all areas affected. Measurement of the lesions and photographs (usually under Wood's lamp) are taken at this or subsequent visit. Some offices have computerized systems to measure the area of the lesions. Except for very small lesions, two scores may be calculated to monitor the disease: VASI and VETF. Both scores are used to monitor the progression of the disease and the effect of treatment.

The VASI score is an estimate of the body's depigmentation by area of the body and is fairly easy to perform (A detailed explanation of how to calculate the score is in the Fall 2011 newsletter of Vitiligo Support International).

The VETF score is used in clinical research but may not be used by a practicing physician. The VETF includes the extent of vitiligo lesions, plus a 0-4 scale of depigmentation, and a 3-unit scale for whether the lesions are stable or spreading.

Tests and referrals will vary depending on the physician's certainty of the diagnosis and of any suspected autoimmune disease. These may include:

Tests:

- *CBC and differential*

Measures of overall health and to rule out anemia

- ***Anti-thyroid peroxidase***

Measures antibodies to a thyroid component; autoimmune thyroid conditions are common among vitiligo patients. Other thyroid tests may be ordered at the initial visit or later.

- ***ANA – Antinuclear Antibody***

ANA – Antinuclear Antibody. Indicates the presence of any autoimmune disease.

- ***Folate and B-12***

Low serum levels of these vitamins are often found among vitiligo patients.

- ***25-Hydroxy-Vitamin D.***

As vitiligo patients are told to avoid the sun, vitamin D levels are often low.

Other

Skin biopsy of the lesion and normal skin. Confirms the diagnosis. Used often when diagnosis is not certain or in very early cases.

Referral for eye exam to check for uveitis.

Referral for ear exam if hearing is suspected to be affected by vitiligo.

3. Vitiligo Appearance

Vitiligo, the first patch

Vitiligo usually develops first on sun-exposed areas of the skin, such as hands, feet, arms, face and lips. Patches are also often seen in areas that tend to experience rubbing, impact, or other trauma, such as underarms, skin fold, the hands, arms, and places where bones are close to the skin surface, such as shins. Sometimes hair over the white patches is white.

A macule is a flat, discolored patch on the skin that is not raised. Most macules – such as birthmarks – are darker than the skin. In vitiligo, the discolored spot is lighter that the surrounding skin. In light-skinned individuals, the patch isn't noticed right away – often not until tanning of the unaffected skin makes the patches show up. It is much more noticeable in persons with dark or tanned skin.

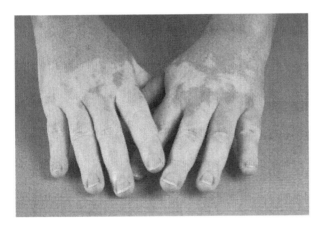

The patch usually has an irregular border. Sometimes there is a sharp edge between the patch and the surrounding skin; other times there is a lighter center spreading to a darker edge. In a small percentage of the time there is a red border, which may or may not be raised.

Eventually most patches turn white, which leaves a chalky white color or sometimes it is light pink from blood circulating beneath thin skin.

In most instances the skin feels the same and there is no pain. Often the patch itches when it first appears and later, if it expands. An exception is with inflammatory vitiligo, which has a raised red rim and persistent itchy skin that is often dry and scaly. Inflammatory vitiligo is very rare, estimated to be less than 1% of all vitiligo patients.

Further patches

For some people, the first patch is all there is. It may even become repigmented later. These cases are rare. For most of those with vitiligo, the first patch expands and other patches appear. Researchers have described several patterns that may occur.

Focal
One or more patch is in a specific area of the body (This describes a point in the disease that may later progress to another type).

Segmental
The patches stop at the midline; if more than one area of the body is involved the patches may be on different sides of the body. Often the number and size of the patches develop rapidly for a year or two but then stabilize. Only rarely does this pattern later change to a generalized pattern.

Mucosal
The patches occur only in mucous membranes such as the lips and inside the mouth, nose, genital, and rectal areas.

Generalized
The generalized patterns are often symmetrical, appearing in the same area on each side of the body at the same time. More often than not, the generalized patterns go through periods of stabilization but then become active again later. This is the most common of the patterns. This pattern is often categorized further to include:

Acrofacial
Patches occur away from the torso. Most often the face and hands but also include the head, and feet.

Vulgaris
Patches are scattered all over the body. It's often called a shower pattern. This term is going out of favor and is included in generalized vitiligo by many.

Mixed
Descriptions of affected areas do not always fit a tidy category. Acrofacial and vulgaris vitiligo may occur in combination, or segmental and acrofacial vitiligo and/or vulgaris.

Universal
The body has no skin pigment, or almost none.

Additional patch characteristics:

Some of the patches have shapes or locations that have been related to actual or assumed causes of the depigmentation:

Koebner's phenomenon
Heinrich Koebner found that some of his psoriasis patients would develop new lesions after trauma to the skin. The new lesions were indistinguishable from older lesions. The appearance of lesions as a result of trauma is now called Koebner's phenomenon.

Koebner's occurs in 20-60% of vitiligo patients. The wide range of estimates is caused by the different questions asked of patients to assess new patches. Trauma can be from many sources including wounds, friction, burns (including sunburn), allergic reactions on the skin, radiation therapy and pressure. It may happen more often during an active phase of the disease.

Blaschko pattern

Sometimes the pattern of vitiligo patches in segmental vitiligo follows Blaschko's lines. The lines are usually invisible but become visible in several skin conditions. The pattern of the lines varies by their location: as in "V" shaped lines in the back, or waves or swirls on the trunk. The lines are believed to be related to genetic differences between cells that occur during the embryonic period. The lines are fairly consistent between people; these lines also found among many animal species.

Dermatomal pattern

In segmental vitiligo the skin patches often follow the path of spinal nerve roots.

Blue Vitiligo

Blue-gray coloring of vitiligo patches occur when there's no melanin in the skin cells but scavenging macrophages, the large white blood cells that clean up debris, have swallowed up melanin or melanosomes, giving the skin some color.

4. Age of onset

Vitiligo may occur at any age, from newborn to the elderly. About half of reported cases are of those under 20 years old. Some have estimated only 5% or so begin after age 40.

How does Vitiligo differ by the age group affected?

Esfandiarpour and Farajzadeh's study (2012) of a consecutive group of new patients at a dermatology practice in Iran found 825 patients with vitiligo. Of the total, 54 or 6.5% had their first vitiligo patch after age 50. Compared with the patients whose condition developed when they were younger, the older onset group displayed greater prevalence of leukotrichia (white hair above the patches) and of Koebler phenomenon (white patches associated with trauma).

15

Studies of young children have shown them to be more likely to have the segmental pattern of vitiligo.

5. Other organs affected by vitiligo

Melanin is scattered throughout the body in almost every organ. In vitiligo patients, the eyes and ears are often affected.

Eyes
Usually when their eyes are examined, vitiligo patients have normal acuity but more than half will have abnormal ocular findings, the most serious – found in 5-7% of patients – is uveitis, affecting the iris or retina/choroid or both. Uveitis is a major cause of blindness worldwide.

There is melanin in the iris, the colored part of the eye; the more melanin, the darker the eye appears. In vitiligo, the color doesn't change but almost half of the melanin may be lost.

Melanin is also present in the choroid, a vascular layer at the back of the eye. The melanin is thought to absorb light and prevent its scattering and causing cloudy vision. The choroid also provides fluid and nutrients to the retina. In vitiligo, the choroid is often depigmented in a striped pattern. Those with highly depigmented choroid often complain of night blindness.

Ears
Hearing loss has been documented in many vitiligo patient groups, ranging from 4% to 38% of those studied, and usually graded mild to moderate. Hearing loss is most apparent for the higher frequency sounds in the 4000-8000 Hz range, although some studies found defects in a lower range. The 4000-8000 range is above most of human speech but includes the ability to distinguish some parts of speech, such as the letters s, h, and f. A piano's highest note is 4000 Hz. The average bird sound is 4000 Hz but warblers, sparrows and other common birds sing at 8,000 Hz and above.

The hearing defect is assumed to be associated with damage to the melanocyte-like intermediate cells of the stria vascularis and of the potassium rich fluid, endolymph; they produce as well as the free melanin they release. The link has been established primarily through animal models.

The visual and hearing problems of most vitiligo patients is much less than those experienced by patients having one of several syndromes that include white skin patches and disorders of hearing and vision. Below are two, one thought to be an autoimmune disease and the other an inherited one.

Vogt-Koyanagi-Harada (VKH) Syndrome
In this condition, melanocytes of the skin, eyes, covering of the brain and spinal cord, and the inner ear are attacked. The condition generally appears in four stages:

- It begins with total body symptoms like the flu, with headache and neck stiffness and sensitivity to noise.
- It's then followed by blurred vision caused by uveitis of the front and back of the eye; sometimes retinal detachments
- A few months later, depigmented choroid at the back of the eye, vitiligo, alopecia (loss of hair in patches), and poliosis (white patches of hair) occurs.
- Patients may have chronic uveitis bouts in later years.

Because of the first symptoms, the cause of VKH was thought to be infectious. Currently it is defined as an autoimmune condition that may sometimes have an infectious trigger. Genetics may also be involved, as patients are predominantly those with darker skin.

Waardenburg syndrome
Waardenburg syndrome is really a group of at least six inherited conditions, one of many with skin, eye and ear involvement. Inheritance is usually (90%) autosomal dominant, so just one parent is needed to pass it on to a child. So many genes are affected however, that even within families, different levels of the

condition are expressed. Hearing loss ranges from minimal to profound and may affect just one ear or both. Hearing impairment is present at birth. This syndrome was discovered primarily as the patients sometimes have eyes of different colors, two colors in the same eye, or brilliant blue eyes. The hairs are those of partial albinism – very pale but not without color.

Chapter 2: The Skin from Top to Bottom

To understand Vitiligo, a good place to start is the basic vocabulary and anatomy of the skin.

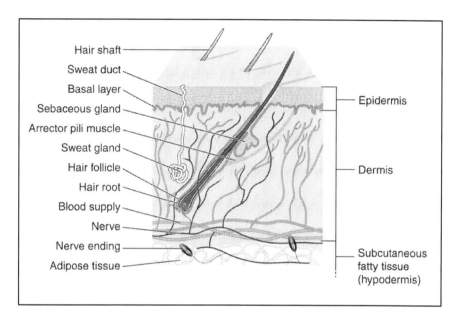

1. Skin Layers

The skin has multiple layers. Starting from the top layer and going to the bottom, interior layer, there are:

Epidermis

The epidermis is the outer or top layer of skin and has four to five sub layers depending upon skin thickness.

Basal cell layer
One row of small cells, called basal cells, lines the bottom layer of the epidermis. These cells are constantly dividing and as each

19

cell divides, one cell is pushed up and the other cell remains to divide again. This migration continues as older and older cells are pushed through the basal layer, then through the other layers of the epidermis to the surface of the skin where they are sloughed off.

Scattered among the basal cells are melanocytes and Merkel cells. Melanocytes produce melanin, the pigment responsible for overall skin color as well as freckles, age spots, and birthmarks. Merkel cells are associated with the nervous system and allow us to feel light touch and distinguish shapes and textures. Both melanocytes and Merkel cells may become malignant and be transformed into aggressive cancers.

Squamous cell layer
This layer contains maturing basal cells, which are now called keratinocytes. The keratinocytes manufacture keratin, which is a tough protective protein for the skin (Nails and hair also contain keratin).

Langerhans cells are found in this layer. These cells arise from the bone marrow and are specialized white blood cells. It's believed these cells recognize antigens and regulate the skin's immune response through interaction with T-cells, the white blood cells that protect against infection.

Stratum granulatum
This is a very thin layer in which the keratinocytes flatten and lose their nuclei. Keratin and waterproofing lipids are organized into tough, durable material.

Stratum lucidim
This thin layer is found only where the skin is thickest, as on the soles of feet and palms of hands. It is thought to reduce the friction between the granulatum layer and the top layer of the epidermis, the stratum corneum.

20

Stratum corneum

This top layer of dead keratinocytes is between 10 and 30 layers thick. The outer layers are rubbed off and replaced from below. In younger people, the entire corneum layer is replaced every month or so, but slows to almost two months in the elderly.

Dermis

The dermis is the thickest layer of the skin. Its functions include supplying nutrients to the epidermis, regulating body temperature, and storing water. This layer has two sublayers.

Papillary layer

This thin vascular layer regulates body temperature by changing blood flow: increased blood flow lowers the body's temperature; decreased flow conserves body heat. The papillary layer also supplies nutrients to the epidermis.

Reticular layer

The reticular layer consists mainly of collagen fibers running in the same direction as the skins surface. The collagen provides strength and elasticity to the skin. Hair follicles, sweat and other glands are located in this layer.

Hypodermis

This layer contains collagen and fat, which insulate the body and protect the inner organs. Blood vessels, nerves, the lymphatic system and hair follicles cross this area.

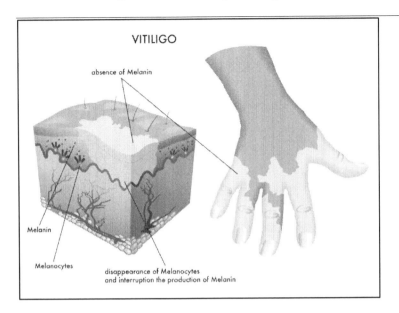

VITILIGO

absence of Melanin

Melanin

Melanocytes

disappearance of Melanocytes
and interruption the production of Melanin

2. Skin Color

Skin color in humans varies throughout the world, primarily depending upon the amount of ultraviolet light the population experiences. Why?

The short evolutionary story is: scientists think that as our ancestors left the African rain forest for the hotter, open grasslands, they lost their heavy body hair and developed sweat glands and darker skin. Darker skin provided long-term survival of the species by protecting the body's supply of folic acid from being destroyed by ultraviolet rays of the sun. Folic acid is one of the essential B vitamins. Without it, adults develop serious blood and organ diseases, become confused and depressed, men are less fertile, and newborns have serious neurological conditions. Darker skin also protected the skin against ultraviolet rays, but as most of the rays' effects – damage to sweat glands and skin cancer – occur after reproduction, it does not affect the species' survival.

As humans migrated to areas away from the equator, dark skin posed a negative side effect as the weaker sunlight caused insufficient vitamin D to be produced by the skin. Vitamin D is essential for forming and maintaining bone growth and structure, and is important in the immune system, muscle strength and overall cell growth and differentiation – all-important for early human survival. Vitamin D is present in useful amounts in just a few foods such as fatty fish, animal livers, and some mushrooms. So the skin paled and vitamin D production increased and all was well.

3. Skin pigments

The color of skin is determined by the type and amount of three pigments: melanin, hemoglobin, and carotene.

Hemoglobin
The hemoglobin in red blood cells circulating in the capillaries gives a pinkish or blue tint to people with pale skin. Pinkish when oxygenated; bluish when not. These colors are evident only among persons with pale skin.

Carotene
Carotene is a fat-soluble molecule that comes from plant sources. It is yellow/red pigment and leaks into the skin from circulating blood. Usually, carotene is not visible in the skin unless a person has pale skin and eats a lot of carrots. Carotene is transformed in the intestine to Vitamin A. This vitamin is essential for cell functions that form and maintain the skin, teeth, bones, soft tissue and mucous membranes, vision, and the immune system. Low vitamin A results in hyperkeratosis (increased thickness of the stratum granulatum and stratum corneum) – with thickened outer layers of the skin, which may be localized or widespread thick white layers of dead skin. Low vitamin A can also cause the cornea of the eye to become opaque and is a common cause of blindness worldwide.

Melanin

This pigment is produced in the skin by melanocytes in the basal layer; about 10% of basal cells are melanocytes. The melanocytes are located in the single cell basal layer and are each connected by their dendrites (finger-like projections) to about 40 keratinocytes (They are also associated with one Langerhans cell).

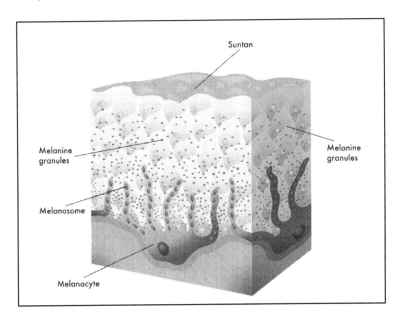

Shape of melanocytes showing melanosomes inside and melanin granules moving toward the skin's surface.

Melanin is produced by cigar-shaped melanosomes; organelles within the melanocytes. Melanosomes are then transported to the keratinocytes where they locate themselves above skin cell nuclei to protect against damaging UV rays.

In addition to being in the basal layer of the skin, melanocytes are also found at hair roots (Melanocytes are also in the eyes, ears and brain)

There are two types of melanin: eumelanin and pheomelanin.

Eumelanin is a pigment that ranges from a tan to black color. Eumelanin reflects and absorbs UV radiation and protects the skin from the effects of the sunrays or tanning booths. Eumelanin is the pigment in gray hair if all other pigments are absent.

Pheomelanin is a reddish-brown pigment. Pheomelanin is responsible for red hair and freckles as well as the color of lips, nipples and areas of genitalia.

4. Scales of skin color

Scientists have devised numerous scales to describe color variations seen in human skin. One scale – Luschan's – offered 36 shades, the first 14 of which are of pinks and blues. In dermatology, these shades have been compressed to six skin types on the Fitzpatrick scale, which is the scale used most often today. These also describe skin and eye color and the skin's response to the sun.

I. Pale white skin; blond or red hair; blue eyes; freckles; burns – never tans

II. White skin; blond or red hair; blue, green or hazel eyes; usually burns – sometimes slight tan

III. Creamy white skin; any hair or eye color; occasional mild burn – tans uniformly

IV. Moderate brown skin, known as a Mediterranean skin tone; rarely burns – always tans well

V. Dark brown, known as a Middle Eastern skin tone; very rarely burns – tans very easily

VI. Deeply pigmented dark brown to black; never burns – tans very easily

What causes these variations in color?

Skin color variation is determined by melanin in the skin but not just by the absolute number of melanocytes. Melanocytes are scattered throughout each person's body in different concentrations but when the forearms of the body are compared, most European skin types have 1,000 to 1,500 melanocytes per square millimeter and darker skin types have 2,000 to 2,500.

Some of the difference in skin color is in the type of melanin produced by the melanosomes. The more eumelanin, the darker the skin. Then there are differences in the number of melanosomes within each melanocyte and their size. Melanosomes in dark skin are twice as long as in white skin and are transferred to skin cells individually and well distributed. In white skin, the more round melanosomes are transferred in clumps and are less uniformly distributed.

Chapter 3: Some Other White Patches

Vitiligo is one of numerous conditions known as leukoderma, from the Latin for 'white skin'. What follows are descriptions of some of the others. A few like albinism may be easily distinguished from vitiligo but others are not. Individuals are warned not to self-diagnose vitiligo as the lesion may be from an entirely different condition.

Albinism
The most widespread of the leukoderma conditions is ocular cutaneous albinism (OCA). This condition is present at birth and affects the melanin of the skin, hair, and retina. Persons with OCA appear extremely pale but some acquire some pigmentation of the skin as they age. Their eyes may be pale blue or red.

OCA is an autosomal recessive inherited condition, so both parents have to have the same affected gene. More than one mutation has been implicated in the condition but they all involve mutations of the gene TYR that controls tyrosinase, a catalyst necessary for the production of melanin. Histology of the skin reveals that melanocytes exist but they have little or no melanin in them.

Piebaldism
Piebaldism, like albinism, is present at birth. The eyes are not affected. The skin patches are similar to those of generalized vitiligo and are symmetrical when present on the trunk and near the elbows and knees. They may be totally depigmented, be uniformly hypopigmented, or be depigmented patches containing circles of normal skin. The most recognizable feature of piebaldism, present in 80 - 90%, is a midline patch in the front of the scalp topped with white hair; sometimes the patch is large enough to also affect the eyebrow and eyelashes on one side. The skin patches differ from vitiligo in that they are stable.

Piebaldism is an autosomal dominant genetic condition, so only one parent with the gene is needed for a child to be affected. There are multiple mutations that cause piebaldism; most are of the KIT gene that involves melanocyte migration and multiplication during embryonic development. Histology of the skin reveals that melanocytes don't exist in the depigmented patches but do in those that are hypopigmented.

Rare syndromes associated with piebaldism—Woolf's and Waardenburg's syndromes – involve various degrees of skin depigmentation, plus the eyes and ears are affected.

Chemical Leukoderma (also called contact leukoderma)
Chemical leukoderma may occur at any age, except it is not present at birth. The initial patch may appear to be a patch signaling vitiligo – a clear white patch – or it may appear as a spattering of small, pea-sized patches. When seen under Wood's lamp, the white patches usually don't luminesce as brightly as in vitiligo.

Chemical leukoderma is caused by exposure to chemicals that either directly or indirectly cause the death of melanocytes. Patients usually have no history of vitiligo or autoimmune diseases themselves or in their families. Occupations in industries where this occurs include rubber, leather, plastic, printing, detergent and photography. Consumers are also affected by hair dyes, lipstick, eyeliner, sprayed perfumes and deodorant, and adhesives. Women are affected in India by azo dyes painted on their feet; in South Asia, women are affected by the adhesive binding bindi, a decorative dot to their foreheads. An American woman was affected by Vicks VaporRub. Phenol and catechol derivatives are often the culprits but a long list of other chemicals have also been implicated (Appendix A).

Prevalence of occupational exposure to these chemicals has been highest in developing countries. Confusion of this condition with

28

vitiligo may account for the high prevalence of vitiligo often reported in the literature for these areas.

While the first patch has been shown to be directly linked to a specific chemical, about 25% of patients later have additional patches in unexposed areas, which form after exposure is stopped. Partial repigmentation sometimes occurs. Because the involved chemicals do not universally affect everyone, and because of the spreading of the lesions to other parts of the body, it is theorized that the affected patients have fragile melanocytes or some other predisposing condition.

Nevus depigmentosus

"Nevus" usually means a birthmark. In this instance, about 70% of patches of nevus depigmentosus are present at birth and most of the remaining were discovered before age three. Most children have just one patch, which can be small and lightly pigmented or large and totally white and resemble vitiligo. Hair of the patches is not pigmented. About a quarter of patients have more than one patch. Multiple patches may appear in a segmental pattern (on one side of the body). Patches are common on the back, buttocks, face and neck, as well as on the hands and feet.

Histology studies differ in that some state that there is no change in the number of melanocytes and others that melanocytes are severely reduced. All agree that the number of melanosomes is greatly reduced. The patients with segmental patterns give rise to the theory that the melanocytes are damaged during formation of the embryo.

Pityriasis Alba

This condition affects 2-5% of children, usually beginning at ages 6 to 12 years but it can affect adults into their 40s. The patches are associated with eczema and allergies. The condition is self-healing; patches may disappear then recur. At first the patches are raised and pink but become pale or white and flat. The patches don't tan and burn easily. They may become flaky, especially in low humidity. The patches are usually on the face, upper chest and back, and upper arms. They can range from tiny to as large as eight inches.

Histology shows fewer and tiny melanosomes and plugged or irregular hair follicles.

Tinea versicolor
Patches for tinea versicolor can be any color from dark brown to white. The patches have a sharp edge, may be numerous, and may grow together. The white patches, if not scaly, look similar to vitiligo and don't tan. The cause is a yeast common on human skin that runs amok. It's most common in teenage boys and men. It runs in some families. It's easily treated (often with dandruff shampoo) but the color changes may remain for some time. It often occurs in hot, moist climates and can be related to immunity and hormone changes. Studies have shown that cell-mediated immunity may be lowered in some cases, with lymphocyte T cells not able to combat the infection. The skin gives a copper yellow luminescence under a Wood's lamp. Skin scraping shows the yeast cells under the microscope.

Tuberous Sclerosis
Tuberous sclerosis is a condition in which non-cancerous tumors grow throughout the body – on the skin, in the brain, heart, lungs, and eyes. The disease can be inherited but usually arises from a spontaneous genetic mutation in about one of every 6,000 births. The condition can run from mild to severe and is characterized in severe cases by intellectual disabilities, seizures, and elevated skin growths (look like bubbly foam or caviar) of the face. Organ damage is caused by the growths expanding and calcifying. Often the first suggestion of the disease is one or more white spots on the skin in the shape of a leaf from an ash tree. The leaf-like image may be present in the newborn; 80% of them appear before the first year (Of course not all leaf-shaped white spots have anything to do with tuberous sclerosis!)

Hansen's disease (Leprosy)

Hansen's disease is a bacterial disease. About 95% of the population has a natural immunity against the disease, which is very rare in the US (100-200 cases a year) but still persists in other parts of the world, with about 200,000 new cases per year. The early skin patches of leprosy are pale but not characteristic of vitiligo. The patches are usually not white and patients have lost the feeling of touch, heat, and pain. There is vitiligo in 10% of patients with later stages of one form of leprosy – the lepromatous or bulbous form.

In the parts of the world where leprosy was widespread there has been great fear and loathing of its victims throughout history. Victims and their families were shunned. This fear still exists in many places and has included vitiligo in its discriminated leprosy population. Not only the white patches of vitiligo but also the language itself has been at fault. In India, for example, the name for vitiligo is "white leprosy".

Chapter 4: Causes and Triggers of Vitiligo

Many theories have existed to explain vitiligo.

1. Genetics

It has been long known that there was some genetic basis for vitiligo, and that the strength of the genetic connection was weaker for vitiligo than for albinism and piebaldism. For example, monozygotic twins share almost all genetic material but have just a 23% chance of both having vitiligo.

Researchers continue to fill in the genetic story and this research is still ongoing. This research is important as each gene or segment of a gene that is linked to vitiligo can point to a chemical or a process that could result in a new approach for treating the disease.

On June 14, 1990, newspapers heralded the discovery of the mutated TYR gene as being responsible for the most severe type of albinism (Type 1A). This mutation causes almost total absence of tyrosinase, which is essential for converting tyrosine to produce melanin.

Mutations of the TYR gene were later linked to patients with generalized vitiligo.

On April 12, 2007, newspapers again announced an important research result. The Human Genome Project studied 656 people with strong family histories of vitiligo and autoimmune diseases. The first gene linking vitiligo to autoimmune diseases was confirmed: NALP1. This gene helps control the body's immune response. (Spritz, 2013)

Subsequently, genetic studies have linked mutations of at least 35 additional loci to vitiligo – all involved in either the chemical production of melanin or in immune responses (Loci are precise chemical addresses within a gene on a chromosome).

2. Autoimmunity

The immune system recognizes pathogens and disables them. Autoimmunity occurs when the body's immune system attacks its own tissues. Early studies of vitiligo patient population found that many vitiligo patients (25-30%) had a recognized autoimmune disease – plus autoimmune diseases were much more common in their families than in the general population.

The body has at least two immunological mechanisms for disabling pathogens:

- B cells (a type of white blood cells) produce antibodies against pathogens.
- T cells recognize and kill pathogens.

In vitiligo, elevated circulating antibodies against many different melanocyte components have been found. Studies have also shown a correlation between some of the antibodies and the amount of depigmentation. Levels of antibodies have been found to be an indicator of recent advancing or stable disease. These antibodies from vitiligo patients have been shown to eliminate melanocytes in the test tube and they depigment human skin transplanted to mice. Questions have been raised about whether the antibodies are evidence that they destroy melanocytes or if they simply occur in reaction to high levels of melanocyte antigens destroyed by other means.

The other mechanism, T cells armed against pathogens, is a little complicated. Called cell-mediated immunity, this system involves special cells called T-cells within the lymphatic system. T-cells are small white blood cells formed in the bone marrow, which mature in the thymus gland (The thymus gland is located in the chest above the heart). There are two types of T-cells, killer and helper cells. The helper cells are involved in target selection – identifying which pathogens the killer cells will attack. And the killer cells kill the pathogen. In the case of vitiligo, the theory is that T-cells are somehow aimed at melanocytes. Activated T-cells against melanocytes have been found at the rims of vitiligo patches and in circulating blood of vitiligo patients.

3. Chemical

Chemically-triggered leukoderma is discussed with "other white patches" as most of the depigmented areas are directly caused by a known chemical irritant, most patients do not go on to experience patches in unexposed areas, and the patients and their families do not have a high percentage of associated autoimmune diseases (Ezzeldine et al., 2012).

4. Neurological

Toxins released by nerve endings have been theorized to be a major cause of segmental vitiligo as the patches closely follow the distribution of a spinal nerve. The toxin theory is supported by case reports of depigmented skin occurring just after a nerve injury (R Yaghoobi et al., 2011).

5. Weak melanocytes

Another theory is that melanocytes are innately defective. While normal melanocytes perform destruction of DOPA and dopachrome, these weak melanocytes cannot and are destroyed by them.

6. Oxidative stress

The production of melanin produces chemicals which when they are metabolized results in hydrogen peroxide, which is toxic to melanocytes. Under normal conditions the enzyme catalase breaks down the hydrogen peroxide into harmless molecules, protecting the melanocytes.

In vitiligo, there is often a shortage of catalase, leading to the death of melanocytes. There is a gene, CAT, which regulates the production of catalase; some studies have shown links of the CAT gene to vitiligo, others have not (Schallreuter et al., 1991).

7. Other triggers

Interviews with patients and their families about events that occurred within a few months of the vitiligo patch first occurring have shown some consistency in identifying severe sunburn, stress, and hormones of puberty and pregnancy as being triggers. Other triggers include periods of poor nutrition, GI infections, and hard knocks to the head. An imbalance of zinc and copper has also been mentioned.

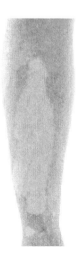

Chapter 5: Associated Illnesses and Conditions

1. Skin Cancer

It would seem reasonable to assume that vitiligo patients would be susceptible to high rates of skin cancer – after all, albino patients have a very high risk. However, vitiligo patients do not. There have been small studies showing increased skin cancers in patients undergoing long term PUVA treatments, but most studies have shown vitiligo patients to have a lower risk than the rest of the population. One reason is thought to be genetics: the same gene that increases the risk of having vitiligo reduces the risk of having melanoma. But the reason for lower non-melanoma skin cancers is still being studied (Teulings, 2013).

A lower risk does not mean that there is no risk of skin cancer. Patients are urged to avoid sunburn and prolonged sun exposure and to use sunscreen and protective clothing. Sunburn can also be a trigger for vitiligo itself and flare-ups.

2. Autoimmune conditions associated with Vitiligo

Vitiligo is considered to be one of the autoimmune diseases – diseases in which the body's immune system attacks a part of itself. About a third of persons with vitiligo also have one or more additional autoimmune disease and these other autoimmune diseases are also present in their relatives. Persons with generalized vitiligo are much more likely than those with segmental (unilateral) vitiligo to have another autoimmune disease (Kutlubay, 2012).

The associated diseases and their frequency differ in reported studies of large groups. This could be from different patient populations (age, stage of disease), geographic areas (different genetic profile), and the range of diagnostic studies performed by a practitioner. Those conditions mentioned most frequently are described below. One reason for describing them is to illustrate the soup of interconnections between and among these conditions with vitiligo. They have so many things in common; often a genetic or family history, a triggering event, and an immune response that creates odd or harmful tricks on the body. It's also important to know about these conditions to be able to provide your physician with a good family history.

Thyroid conditions

Thyroid conditions are the more common of the autoimmune conditions associated with vitiligo. Studies of populations of vitiligo patients find 10-20% have a clinical thyroid condition. Thyroid hormones regulate metabolism, body temperature, heart rate, muscle strength, and renewal of body cells.

Hashimoto's thyroiditis (hypothyroid condition)
Hashimoto's thyroiditis is an autoimmune disease, which involves the destruction of the thyroid gland. The immune process is mediated by T- cells (white blood cells produced in the thymus gland) that cause inflammation and destruction of the gland. The patients' blood contains antibodies against thyroid proteins, thyroperoxidase and thyroglobulin. Patients with this disease also may have any one of the conditions in this section plus multiple sclerosis.

The pituitary releases large amounts of thyroid stimulating hormone (TSH) to try to make the thyroid gland work – thus the condition is often diagnosed by testing for TSH levels.

Symptoms include fatigue, depression, intolerance to cold, and being sleepy. Untreated, the disease can be fatal. Treatment is with thyroid hormones.

Graves' disease (hyperthyroid condition)

Graves' disease is unusual in that the immunoglobulins involved – thyroid stimulating immunoglobulins (TSIs) – don't attack the thyroid gland. Instead, they mimic the pituitary gland's production of thyroid stimulating hormone (TSH) and cause the thyroid gland to overproduce thyroid hormones. As there are plenty of circulating thyroid hormones, the pituitary gland decreases TSH production.

Symptoms include a thyroid gland twice the normal size, protruding eyes, fatigue, and weight loss despite healthy food intake, rapid heart, and muscle weakness. The tissue around the eyes swells and may push the eyes forward.

There are lab tests for TSIs but the diagnosis is usually made based upon symptoms, TSH levels (they are low), and thyroid hormone levels (they're high).

Addison's disease (cortisone reduction)

Addison's disease is caused by a decrease in the hormones released by the adrenal gland (The adrenal gland sits above the kidney). Adrenal hormones regulate sugar, sex hormones, sodium and potassium, immune response, and response to stress. About 80% of Addison's disease in adults is of autoimmune origin. The disease is usually recognized after much of the adrenal gland is gone and its production of cortisone decreases to the point that symptoms appear. Common symptoms include weight loss with low appetite, muscle weakness, extreme fatigue, low blood pressure, and sometimes darkening of the skin. Can be fatal if untreated. Treatment is replacement corticosteroids. Addison's disease is associated with every other disease listed in this section.

Pernicious anemia (B12 absorption defect)

In the stomach, parietal cells produce a protein called intrinsic factor. Intrinsic factor allows vitamin B12 to be absorbed. The bone marrow needs vitamin B12 to make healthy red blood cells (RBCs). In pernicious anemia, the body's immune system attacks the parietal cells and decreases absorption of B12. The result is that the defective RBCs are often so large that they can't escape the bone marrow, and the ones that are in circulation perform poorly.

Symptoms are fatigue, which increases as the disease progresses; pale skin; cold hands and feet; enlarged heart; and nerve damage. The condition used to be fatal, but now, if diagnosed, it can be treated with B12 pills or injections. Most patients with this condition are adults or elderly and often of northern European stock.

Associated autoimmune conditions include Addison's disease, Grave's Disease, thyroiditis, and systemic lupus erythematosus.

Diabetes mellitus (Type1)

Insulin is made in the pancreas by beta cells in the islets of Langerhans. Most cells of the body get energy from glucose. Insulin helps glucose get into the cells. In diabetes mellitus Type 1, the body's immune system attacks the beta cells and other antigens of the islets. As insulin decreases, cells start using the body's fat and muscle for energy. The glucose stays circulating in the blood. At some point, the glucose levels rise to the point that the kidneys can't simply return the glucose to the blood so they excrete it – along with a lot of water and minerals. Patients begin to urinate frequently, feel thirsty, lose weight, and have blurry vision. Treatment is insulin injections and dietary restrictions.

Autoimmune conditions associated with Type 1 diabetes include thyroid conditions, celiac disease, vitiligo, pernicious anemia, and Addison disease.

Type 1 patients are usually diagnosed from childhood to early adulthood. Now, however, Type 1 is being found in older adults who started out as Type 2 patients. In Type 2 diabetes (which is 90-95% of all diabetes patients), the pancreas produces insulin, but not enough. It is associated with obesity, a diet high in fat and certain carbohydrates, and a sedentary lifestyle.

Systemic lupus erythematosus (multi-organ condition)

In systemic lupus erythematosus (SLE), the body's immune system may attack any major organ of the body. Studies have shown that antibodies may be present many years before the disease is apparent. About half of patients have a raised, red butterfly-shaped skin inflammation over the cheeks and nose, sometimes spreading to the forehead. Others begin with discoid lupus, a more severe skin inflammation. About 5-10% of the skin conditions develop into SLE.

About 90% of patients are women, usually aged 10-40. African Americans and Asians are more likely than others to have the condition. Patient symptoms will depend upon the organs involved: joint pain, fever, hair loss, extreme sensitivity to sun, headaches, vision and psychiatric symptoms, coughing up blood from lungs, circulatory problems in the hands, etc. Patients are at a higher risk for blood cancers than the general population.

Family histories often include other autoimmune diseases. Sunlight may be a trigger. In about 5% of cases, medications for another disease are the triggers – about forty drugs have been identified. Symptoms abate with withdrawal of the drugs.

Treatments are aimed at reducing inflammation and damping the immune response. Symptoms may wax and wane over the life of the patient. Lupus is a very serious condition; the death rate of patients with the diagnosis is twice that of the general populations.

Psoriasis

In psoriasis, the immune system thinks skin cells are pathogens and attack them. The attack signals new skin cells to develop. These new skin cells develop in just a few days instead of the four weeks or so for normal skin cells. Skin cells pile up in the affected area and are not sloughed off. A patient may have just a few red or white patches of psoriasis or almost all the skin may be involved.

Psoriasis is most common in ages 15-30 and 50-60 and affect about 2% of the total population. Whites have a higher incidence than those with darker skin. About a third of patients have a family history of psoriasis. Triggers include emotional or physical stress (as recovery from an illness). The condition may worsen with alcohol, smoking, obesity, infections, injury to the skin, hot water, or changes in climate.

About 30% of patients also have arthritis. The disease is chronic and can be troublesome to treat. Treatments include a long list of local, systemic, and phototherapy options. Research is focused at blocking one of the steps involved in the immune response.

Alopecia areata (hair loss)

Alopecia areata (AA) usually begins as a bald spot or two, usually on the scalp. In 1-2% of patients it can spread to the entire scalp or even include all body hair, including eyelashes and nose hair. The process may hurt or tingle. Gray hair is not affected.

In the normal hair growth cycle there is a long (4-10 year) period where the hair is produced. Then there is a short (2-3 week) period where the hair follicle regresses, followed by a 1-3 month resting phase. During the resting stage, the follicle is about 5% of its normal size.

In AA, immune cells (mostly T lymphocytes) swarm into and around the hair follicle causing the follicle to shift prematurely into a resting phase. The immune cells spread out in a fairly circular pattern and enlarge the affected area. The follicles remain otherwise healthy in AA and continually try to grow hair. As long as the immune cells are there, the follicles produce just tiny wisps, then cycle back to a resting stage. When there is a marked decrease in immune cells, the follicles will begin to make decent hair even after years and years.

Many patients affected by AA are young and healthy – teens and young adults are the population most often affected. There is often some family history of AA or other autoimmune diseases. Patients may have other autoimmune diseases – hypothyroidism, lupus, and rheumatoid arthritis have been reported.

Most patients have small patches that regrow in a year or so spontaneously. Maybe 10% of patients have more extensive hair loss and about 1% have total body loss of hair. The larger and more aggressive the loss of visible hair, the harder the disease is to treat and may be considered a chronic condition, although spontaneous regrowth years later may still occur. Different therapies may have initial success of 50-90% hair regrowth, but not all the regrowth is cosmetically pleasing for the patient, and regrowth is not permanent much of the time. Treatments include topical/intralesional/systemic corticosteroids, UV and laser therapy, and immunotherapy.

Rheumatoid arthritis

Rheumatoid arthritis (RA) is an autoimmune inflammatory disease in which the synovial membrane of joints is inflamed, is painful, and which over time may deform the joints to the point they cannot move. Inflammation is not limited to joints –

inflamed blood vessels can lead to defects of the skin, nerves, heart, lungs, and brain. The interior or exterior membranes of the heart can be affected.

Patients are often (70%) female. The age group with joint damage is first detected is 30-50 years. A family history of RA increases the risks by 3-9 times. The disease is suspected of having a genetic base, which is sparked by environmental triggers. These triggers include smoking, occupational chemical exposure, infections, dietary, or hormones.

An antinuclear antibody, RA-33, appears in the serum of patients long before symptoms appear. This antibody is also present in systemic lupus erythematosus and mixed connective disease.

Treatment includes over-the-counter anti-inflammatory drugs, corticosteroids and two types of medications called disease modifying anti-rheumatic drugs (DMARDs). DMARDs are of two types – one traditional chemical compounds given in pill form such as methotrexate. The other type, biologic response modifiers – or biologicals – are proteins developed to modify particular spots within the immune reaction. The biologicals are given in a medical office either injections under the skin or IV from one a week to monthly. Often one or two of the non-biologic drugs are given at once, or combined with a biological. Both types of DMARDs are effective but have serious side effects. Corticosteroids and the non-biologicals are affordable under most health plans. The biologicals are expensive running from $2,000 to $15,000 per month.

Inflammatory bowel disease

Inflammatory bowel disease (IBD) may not be an autoimmune disease. About 2% or so of vitiligo patients have inflammatory bowel disease (IBD). There are two major conditions of IBS, Crohn's disease (CD) and ulcerative colitis (UC). They differ in the part of the digestive system affected and how deeply the tissue is damaged: CD affects the lining of the colon and rectum; UC affects deeper structures of the entire digestive tract. Both conditions cause abdominal pain and diarrhea. Family history is a factor in the disease with dozens of genes involved. While IBD patient serum contain antibodies to gut antigens, these antigens may be a reaction to dead cells from inflammation and ulcers caused by accumulation of overactive white blood cells attacking food and organisms in the gut.

IBD is associated with autoimmune diseases, most notably arthritis, psoriasis, and multiple sclerosis. Treatments include immunosuppressive and anti-inflammatory drugs.

Autoimmune polyglandular syndrome

Autoimmune polyglandular syndrome is a rare disease, it is important to geneticists and immunologists because it is the first and only systemic (body-wide) autoimmune disease whose cause has been attributable to a defect in a single gene.

Autoimmune polyglandular syndrome (APS) is a group of diseases in which the immune system attacks the endocrine systems. The syndrome is divided into three separate conditions; they are all treated by replacement hormones.

Type I
Type I APS is the only one of the three types to have one gene responsible for the condition. The AIRE or autoimmune regulator gene regulates production of the protein autoimmune regulator. Found mostly in the thymus, this protein helps the T cells recognize the difference between the body's own cells and the antigens they are supposed to attack. In Type 1APS this protein doesn't help and the T cells begin to sense that some of the endocrine glands are the enemy. The gene is autosomal recessive, requiring both parents to have the gene for their child to be affected.

44

This disease affects children between 5 and 15 years old. And the sequence is hyperparathyroidism, followed in five years by hypothyroidism, followed in another five years by adrenal gland failure. These patients also often have other autoimmune diseases Type 1A diabetes, alopecia, and vitiligo.

Type II

Type II APS affects three times as many women as men; and patients usually begin showing symptoms in their thirties. There is no single gene responsible but about half of patients have a family history of the disease. Years ago it was thought that TB was responsible for the disease but now autoimmunity is thought responsible for the majority of cases.

This disease involves the adrenal gland first, then hyper- or hypo-thyroid condition, followed by Type 1 diabetes.

Type III

Type III APS affects the same population as Type II. The disease starts with hypo- or hyper- thyroid condition but does not involve the adrenal gland. The diagnosis includes the presence of at least one other autoimmune disease, which may be diabetes, premature menopause, pernicious anemia, alopecia, vitiligo, celiac disease or myasthenia gravis

Chapter 6: Management of Vitiligo

Vitiligo has been known for centuries, though often mistaken for a form of leprosy. Given the social stigma that so often occurred, many attempts were made to cover the white patches. Some, like today's methods, were camouflage techniques using tea, bark, and seeds. Others used concoctions of weeds that actually caused the skin to repigment. Some of those "weeds" – like bavachee in India and similar plant-based substances in Egypt and China – contain psoralen which is still a treatment used today.

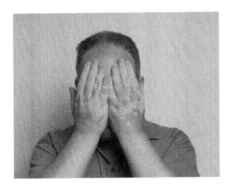

Today's treatment choices depend upon the size, stage, and location/distribution of the patches, the patient's age, and available services in the community. So far, treatments have yet to reach the goal of providing stable, long lasting, repigmented skin, but many are giving good cosmetic results.

Not all of the possible treatments have been described. It would be a futile undertaking as there are so many. Some of the more recent approaches and paths opened by recent research are discussed in the research section.

The options for patients are many and described below.

1. Do nothing

For patients with very light skin and small patches no treatment may be needed as the contrast between the depigmented and pigmented skin is not noticeable or is not bothersome for the patient. Patients are warned that if their skin tans, the patches will be more visible. While some recommend no sunlight at all, some sunlight or artificial light sources are thought to be beneficial in keeping remaining melanocytes functioning.

Patients choosing the "do nothing" option should be informed of the potential advancement of their vitiligo and that delay in treatment may limit their later choices. Most first line treatments need available melanocytes in hair follicles and vitiligo patch margins to work. Patients should also be offered advice for camouflage.

2. Sunscreen

As noted above, sunscreens are helpful in keeping the contrast between pigmented and depigmented skin less noticeable. While the areas of the patches lack melanocytes, reducing the risk of melanoma, other skin cells need this protection. In addition, since sunburn is a known trigger for vitiligo, it needs to be avoided. Some camouflage products used in vitiligo include sunscreen.

Sun protective clothing is also an effective sunscreen. Regular clothing made of tightly woven polyester, nylon, wool, silk and denim are especially good at stopping UV light. Specially manufactured sun-protective garments have the UPF number on the label.

A note of caution

Manufactured nanoparticles are now included in numerous cosmetic products, including foundations and sunscreens. Nanoparticles are tiny particles made from existing chemicals.

They occur in nature from burning; many components of ash are nanoparticles. The size of nanoparticles ranges from 1 to 100 nanometers. For an idea of how small this is – the herpes virus is 100 nanometers in size.

Nanoparticles may or may not act the same way as the original chemical. In cosmetics, they are valued for their ability to provide greater cover with less compound. A future value is the hope that the tiny nanoparticles' ability to penetrate cell walls can be used to treat skin conditions directly instead of by using oral medications.

Concern with nanoparticles has been building as the particles are small enough to pass through cell membranes and some have been found to be toxic. Nanoparticles have been found in the lung from use of aerosol products. Europe now requires that cosmetic labels add "(nano)" to any nanoparticle ingredient. Nanoscale zinc was has been approved for use in European sunscreens, except in sprays and powders. Swedish companies can't market any product containing nanoparticles.

In the US, the FDA issued guidelines in June 1914 addressing nanoparticles in cosmetics. The FDA does not require any premarket proof of cosmetics safety, but does have a list of chemicals that can't be used in them. For now, companies are encouraged to contact the FDA before marketing new products containing nanoparticles and also to contact the FDA regarding test methods and data needed to substantiate product safety.

So, better safe than sorry. Until the safety of any nanoparticle has been adequately determined, vitiligo patients should limit the use of products that contain them as they may use sunscreen more than most people, and may have large areas of skin covered by camouflage products. Be especially wary of products in powder form or aerosols (in spray cans, airbrush, or self-tanning booth) that contain nanoparticles.

Information is still lacking on each product's nanoparticle content. Some manufacturers do not respond to requests for that information. The Wilson Center has attempted to compile a list of cosmetics, which can be seen at www.nanotechproject.org/cpi/. Products that cause shimmering or are advertised to make skin appear lighter are apt to contain nanoparticles.

3. Camouflage

Vitiligo is a chronic condition. A patient may try more than one type of treatment to repigment his/her skin, and each treatment may require several months before seeing results. Many of the patients are young – a time when it's particularly difficult to be different. Camouflage offers temporary coverage for the vitiligo patients during treatment.

Even successful treatments for vitiligo tend not to be permanent. Camouflage is often used to touch up fading skin. Some patients with stable vitiligo retire from medical therapies and use camouflage on and off – maybe using products on their face and hands much of the time and doing other areas only for special occasions. Camouflage has been shown to improve quality of life for those who want them. Children as young as 6 years old have been found capable of applying camouflage independently.

There is a wide variety of products are now available to blend the depigmented skin into that not affected. Some are applied daily as makeup, others provide longer-term skin color.

In the US, health insurance doesn't reimburse for camouflage. In the UK things are different, perhaps because of formal camouflage programs developed there in hospitals during the 1950s and incorporated within its national health system (NHS). There is a free volunteer organization, Changing Faces, which helps patients find products that match their skin and provides instruction on applying it. There is also another organization, The British Association of Skin Camouflage (BASC), which trains several different professionals in skin camouflage techniques. These professionals operate both within the NHS and outside the national system. Basic camouflage products are included as prescription items. The fee per prescription is 8.05£ ($13), but an annual certificate for prescription drugs is available for 104£ ($170) that covers all prescriptions for that year. Also children under 16, children 16-18 if in school, and people 60+ are not charged for any prescriptions. The camouflage products in the regular formulary are: Covermark, Keromask, Dermablend, Dermacolor, and Veil Cover Cream.

Judging from patient reports, in the US a patient often gets little or no help at all from their physician – often not even being told about the products that are available. Camouflage experts can be found in the US in cosmetic departments of national department stores or salons, attached to cosmetic surgery offices, or in private practices.

Dyes
Dyes range from do-it-yourself recipes using food colors (or other natural dyes such as henna) and rubbing alcohol. As long as they are safe for the body, experiments can do no harm – they have been used for centuries. Many find good matching skin color from dyes. The problem with dyes is that they wash away. Henna has a lot of red in it. Browns are often formed using potassium permanganate, indigo carmine, or bismark brown.

Mentioning the word dyes made me remember to be careful using hair dyes. Many hair-coloring products contain phenol and these should be avoided as they can cause depigmentation.

Foundations/concealers
Many creams are available that, with a fixing powder or spray, provide excellent cover for 8 to 16 hours. They are quite resistant to smudging or water. Some are better for swimming pools; a few are better for water sports. Some are better for oily skin, some better for dry. Some are better for lighter or darker shades of skin.

Some have just a few colors (but more can be made by mixing two or different colors) and some have a palette of 200 or more colors. Results are best if color matching can be done in the patient's community. Most products can then be purchased online.

Patient message boards and member chat rooms, such as the one for Vitiligo Support International, are excellent sources for product advice. Some people are happy with regular waterproof makeup products such as Physician's Formula and Makeup Forever for small skin areas. Sephora is a company with many locations in the US that patients recommend for their wide stock of concealers. (I mention product names that repeatedly show up in patient conversations and online reports as shorthand for the type of product – not an endorsement. I was happy when I went on the Sephora site and in the FAQ section someone asked about white spots and was told by another person it was probably vitiligo and to seek medical help.)

Some guidelines and notes for the use of these products:

- To avoid skin infections, these products need to be removed from the face and neck each day and the skin cleaned. Avoid skin cleaners with alcohol or acetone. Body makeup (assuming a thin preparation is used) may be left on for a few days.
- Products made specifically for camouflaging skin conditions are usually free of harmful products. If using other products alone or over camouflage, avoid any chemicals labeled as paraben, urea, or fragrance. **Note**: Also, for now, avoid products containing nanoparticles, which have not yet been found safe as discussed above in the section on sunscreens.
- Products made specifically for camouflage have much more pigment than regular makeup products.
- Lighter skin tones are easier to find colors to match. Some find by using a DHA self-tanning product first provides a better base to work from than the white vitiligo patch.

- Don't forget you have many different colors on your skin. Where the sun hits and where it doesn't are the main differences.
- Be patient, it may take several tries to get the result you are looking for.
- Apply the product in the middle of the vitiligo patch and blend it with a brush, sponge, or finger towards the boundary. This avoids darkening the surrounding skin.
- There are body makeup products that work well. These are usually spray or bottled products and provide a thin cover. The cover can be made more smudge-proof by using a fixing spray.
- Regular makeup can be used over the concealer to match with the rest of the skin. Sometimes using bronzer can give a more natural look. Areas of normal skin can be lightened a little with concealer to match the vitiligo area.
- Some people use spray-on nylons. These products are similar to the "airbrush" type sprays, not self-tanning chemicals. They can be messy to apply ... some do it outside the house.
- For touchups, there are stick forms of camouflage. Colors may be limited. Brands include Erace and Spotstick. There are lip concealers and dyes with cover balms.
- It's handy to have a test kit of the brand of concealers that work for you. You can add some additional realism to the color and use on areas that are of a different color to your main patch.

Microskin

An Australian firm has a product that when dabbed or sprayed onto the skin dries to become a polyurethane film. For someone living in cities where they have stores – right now they're in California and New York in the US –a person's skin color is analyzed by a computer and a dye for the film is compounded. The store experience includes a fee for the analysis and lessons on how to apply the product. They also offer a starter kit ($200; 123£) for people not living near a store.

The film lasts at least a day and people who sleep with it on report that it doesn't come off on the linens. The product blocks sun rays. Product reviews vary. Some are happy and say they don't feel the film while others complain of the color, feel, and look. The firm reports that men are attracted to this technique.

DHA

Many patients use and are happy with sunless tanning solutions containing DHA (dhydroxyacetone). A popular product is Dy-O-Derm. DHA is a carbohydrate usually manufactured from sugar. When dissolved in creams or liquids and applied to the skin, it bonds with amino acids in the corneum layer, that outside layer of dead cells. Before applying the solution, the skin is roughed up to strip the outermost cells off. After applying the solution, a brown color appears within a few hours. Color concentration is related somewhat to the amount of DHA in the preparations which range from 3% to 12% or more.

DHA does not provide a good color match for yellow skin tones.

The color from DHA does not protect the skin from the sun. Some creams and lotions containing DHA include a sunscreen; if they don't, patients need to use their regular sun-safe routine. The DHA product is often not as successful for very dark skin and must be applied only on the depigmented areas, as it will darken the normal surrounding skin. The products take a little practice to apply evenly. Color lasts from a day or two to as long as two weeks before another application is needed.

If the contrast is not too great between depigmented and pigmented skin, some find success using spray-tanning booths at salons and sports centers. Some products dry more quickly than others. A usual warning is to stay out of the sun for a day after application – DHA exposed to sun promotes oxidation, a trigger for vitiligo.

The skin color doesn't stain clothing or linens. It does fade quickly in sweat and ocean water but stays well in fresh water and pools.

Sunless tanning products are available in lotions, creams, and as liquids for spraying. Spraying equipment costs around $100 (62£) and tinted (to avoid overlap in spraying) and clear liquids are available at fairly reasonable costs.

Felt-tip pens
At least one company, Magic Stylo, has semi-permanent ink pens. Patients have found this product useful in covering small areas. The pens have a fine point and have three shades of brown. Skin matching is not as good as for camouflage products but the color is fairly durable, lasting 12-48 hours.

Tattooing
Cosmetic tattooing can be successful in the right hands. Tattooing is an art and not every person providing cosmetic tattooing is an artist. Definitely a buyer beware type of service. Blogs are helpful here. Anyone investing in this service should expect to meet someone in person who's been successfully treated for a similar type of skin and area involved.

In addition to the quality of the art, research is needed to assure the training, proper pigments, and sterility of instruments. New needles and new pigment containers should be opened each time. The practitioner should be licensed (if required) and credentialed by the American Academy of Micropigmentation and Society of Permanent Cosmetics Professionals – or their equivalent.

Patients with vitiligo that have been stable for five years or so can benefit from this semi-permanent procedure. (Tattooing has been reported to cause new patches if vitiligo still active.) There should be no highly pigmented zone around the patch. Patients who tan a lot aren't pleased with the result. Sometimes the skin of vitiligo patients absorbs too much pigment in spots, which may take a long time to fade. In addition, there are scores of conditions that make tattooing a bad idea which need to be discussed with a physician; these include a tendency to scar badly, or who have chronic skin conditions such as psoriasis or chronic infectious disease.

The pigments used are medical grade iron oxide and ground very small. Tattooing is usually done in steps to be sure not to over-pigment the area. Very fine needles are used to push the pigments into the dermis. Results are not permanent. There is some immediate fading, then fading from sun and other stress on the skin. The need for touchups varies; some need annual touchups, others just every two to four years.

Small areas of the face that aren't repigmented any other way are best candidates – such as the lips and the skin circling the lips. Hands are a bit painful to have tattooed and the pigments fade more quickly. The European Dermatology Forum consensus recommends tattooing for lips and nipples only. Young people are cautioned against tattooing with the hope that new treatments now being studied will be effective.

Cost can be a barrier. Depending upon size and difficulty, initial costs range from $1,000 to $3,000 (616 –1848£) or more. Touchups range from $100 to $500 (62- 310£) each visit.

Some folks with vitiligo decorate their patches with regular permanent tattoo art. Cautions again are to avoid tattooing an active vitiligo patch and to avoid infections. Some of the results are quite beautiful.

4. Prescription Medicines

Not all patients will have their vitiligo patches treated successfully. Repigmenting will depend upon how new the disease is when treatment starts, and the size, location, and distribution (focal, generalized, or segmented) of the skin patches

– as well as just plain luck. About 10-20% of patients fully recover their skin color.

Not all dermatologists treat vitiligo: sites of vitiligo organizations advise new patients not to make a doctor's appointment before verifying that there is an option of active treatment for vitiligo if they want it. Some physicians prefer providing information and reassurance concerning the nature of the disease. Patients electing an active treatment should be curious how a physician monitors treatment progress – photographs are essential in tracking the slow progress of many of the treatments. A frank discussion is also needed at the beginning about what the patient and the doctor consider a success – one may consider only 100% repigmenting acceptable while the other's goal may be closer to 50%.

How do you find a physician? You may get referrals from:

- Primary care physician
- Medical school dermatology department
- A satisfied vitiligo patient. This could be someone you know or found through vitiligo support organizations
- The American College of Dermatology has locations of dermatologists in the US but can't make referrals to individual physicians

What are you looking for in a treating physician? Ideally someone who:

- Knows about vitiligo, its potential causes and treatments
- Takes you and vitiligo seriously
- Is confident of your diagnosis
- Has treated 50 or more patients with success in at least 30%
- Is interested in vitiligo, keeps up with newer treatments and research
- Has a Wood's lamp in office
- Has nbUVB in office

- Takes photos of patches to follow treatment outcomes
- Can provide emotional support, advice on diet and sun exposure
- Can be honest about result of treatment both good and bad

Repigmenting may occur as a gradual freckling that starts as tiny dots and finally fills in. Another pattern is for the patch to shrink from the borders to the center. Patterns depend upon healthy melanocytes in hair follicles and on the bordering skin. (That's why skin covered with white hairs is more difficult to treat.)

The numerous treatments described here are not inclusive. This reflects the multiple causes of vitiligo and the lack of success of any one treatment.

Corticosteroids
Corticosteroids suppress the body's immune response and inflammation, both features of vitiligo. Corticosteroids have been used for more than fifty years to treating vitiligo. Side effects of both systemic and topical preparations have limited their use.

Oral corticosteroids are successful in stopping the progression of widespread active vitiligo. Studies have also reported high repigmenting rates in active but not in stable vitiligo.

Strategies to avoid the complications of the oral medications have included using a very low daily dose; starting with a high dose but then lowering doses systematically; or pulsed dosing – giving as low a dose as possible for two days in a row each week. Studies continue. Oral corticosteroid treatments are limited to 2-4 months to avoid serious side effects; the short-term side effects include weight gain (from increased appetite) and mood change or swings. Longer treatment can cause muscle weakness, acne, diabetes, high blood pressure, problems with wound healing and susceptibility to infections – to name a few!

Topical corticosteroids have been successful in stopping the progression of small new vitiligo patches – and are good for repigmenting the skin of the elbows and knees and they work well on dark skin. Now most use calcineurin inhibitors for the face and neck. Some report repigmenting – 30% or so on the legs. Usually a fairly strong corticosteroid is chosen for the body; either limited to 3 months of daily application or cycles of 15 days of treatment/15 days of no treatment for as long as 6 months.

Topical corticosteroids are graded by their effect on the blood vessels in the skin. Grades I to VII range from strongest to the weaker drugs.

- I   Clobetasol diproprionate 0.05% (Temovate)
- II   Fluocinonide 0.05% (Lidex)
- III   Mometasone furoate 0.1% (Elocon ointment)
- IV   Fluocinolone acetonide 0.01-0.2% (Synalar, Synemol, Fluonid)
- V   Triamcinalone acetonide 0.1% (Kenalog, Aristocort cream, lotion
- VI   Prednicarbate 0.05% (Aclovate cream, ointment)
- VII   Hydrocortisone 2.5% (Hytone cream, lotion, ointment); Hydrocortisone 1% (Many over-the-counter brands)

Side effects of topical corticosteroids include streaks that look like stretch marks, skin thinning, or atrophy (feels like the skin has been stretched). To avoid the side effects, calcineurin inhibitors are now often used on the face.

Some of newer Level II corticosteroids such as mometasone furoate and methylprednisolone aceponate have few local and systemic side effects. These preparations are used for treating large areas, for children, and for areas with thin skin (around eyes, genitals).

Calcineurin inhibitors

Topical calcineurin inhibitors are a newer class of non-steroidal, anti-inflammatory drugs now replacing many of the topical corticosteroids. These drugs block calcineurin, which in turn reduces T cells in the vitiligo skin and their production of cytokines. The cytokines kill melanocytes in autoimmune reactions of vitiligo. There is some thought that the calcineurin inhibitors also affect melanocytes in a good way – helping them migrate to depigmented areas of the skin and mature.

If these medications don't work after six weeks, they're usually discontinued. If they don't work, the assumption is that the base cause of the patient's vitiligo was not autoimmunity.

The two inhibitors used in vitiligo treatments are tacrolimus (Protopic) and pimocrolimus (Elidel). These drugs were initially approved for other uses: tacrolimus for moderate to severe eczema and pimocrolimus to reduce rejection in transplant medicine. For treating vitiligo, they provide the equivalent of a Level I corticosteroid.

These medicines work on par with topical corticosteroids (applied twice a day) but without the side effects of the steroid. They work very well on the face, but less well or not at all when used elsewhere. They generally shorten the time needed to show the beginning of repigmenting. Their effectiveness on the legs has been studied and found to be improved by applying them at night and covering them with film, foil, or another barrier.

They don't cause skin thinning or atrophy. When treatment is started, patients report temporary stinging, itching, and burning. More rare side effects have been reported including headache, flu symptoms, and herpes. People with weakened immunity can't use them.

Drinking alcohol while using these drugs causes the face to flush and feel hot. Patients are told to limit sun exposure, and wear sunscreen, although some daily sun is recommended. Protopic is greasy (having a petroleum base) causing some patients not to use it in the morning. Elidel is a creamy preparation. Both are applied in tiny amounts and rubbed into the skin.

The drugs can be used for longer periods than the corticosteroids: they stay at the skin and are not absorbed in any measurable way into the blood stream.

The FDA has a "Black Box" warning for these drugs and their potential for causing lymphomas. Lymphomas have occurred with oral doses of these drugs but have not been reported when applied on the skin.

V-tar

V-tar is a coal tar prescription product that is a water-soluble clear liquid. It also contains natural anti-inflammatory agents, skin conditioners, and antioxidants. V-tar is an early chemical in dermatology – in the 1920's it was used with phototherapy for psoriasis. Some patients have an allergic reaction to the additives in the product.

For vitiligo, the usual 30% solution is applied to the skin once a week and left overnight or for at least six hours. This is a phototoxic drug - sun has to be avoided for the next three days to avoid exaggerated sunburn. Sun or phototherapy is not used at any time in the treatment. The product is safe for children as long as they can be kept safe from the sun. Without sun, the skin surrounding vitiligo patches is not darkened and the repigmentation, which occurs, is done safely.

V-tar is still a product that some insurance companies consider a first line drug before allowing other treatments. It is said to be effective in many patients.

5. Light therapies

PUVA

Light therapy was a treatment of the ancients. In fact, they invented the combined drug + light therapies now in common use. People with vitiligo would make compounds from their "weeds" containing psoralen, spread them on their skin, then stay in the sun. Their first mode was to stay in the sun until the vitiligo patches blistered, but eventually an easier way was found: eat the berries, stay in moderate amounts of sunlight.

A few notes on sunlight. Ultraviolet light, or UV light, is light that reaches the earth but people can't see it. UV light has been divided in UVA, UVB, and UVC.

- UVA: The longer wave, 320-400 nm. This is about 95% of all UV that reaches earth; passes through glass; penetrates the skin deeply; has even distribution during the day; causes ageing of skin and wrinkles and may initiate skin cancers. UVA causes melanin already in the skin to darken.
- UVB: Shorter than UVA, 290-320 nm. Fluctuates by time of day – highest between 10 and 4; causes skin reddening and sunburn. UVB stimulates production of melanin by melanocytes.
- UVC: Shortest of the UV waves, 200-290. Most UVC is absorbed by the ozone and doesn't reach the earth's surface. It is believed that most UVC that hits the skin is absorbed by the upper layer of dead cells. However, UVC is absorbed by organic substances like DNA and this ability lies behind UVC being used to kill microbes.

Modern medicine's light treatment began exactly the same as the ancient's, except psoralen was purified. It is taken orally or applied topically either as a cream or, if much of the body is affected, often in baths. After a wait of 1-2 hours, patients are then placed under UVA lamps, usually with UV ranging from

315-400 nm, peaking at 350 nm. Some physicians skip the UVA step and advise their patients to get some sun on the patches instead.

These modern-day psoralen/light treatments are called PUVA for psoralen UVA light. PUVA can be used to treat generalized and segmental forms of the disease. Patients with darker skin have the best results. About 70% have some repigmenting. All areas of the body except the hands and feet respond well. Treatments can require 1-2 years of 2-3 visits to the doctors' office a week. Complete repigmenting occurs in about 20% of patients. Unfortunately, after all the effort, more than half of patients relapse within a year or two.

Children are treated with caution: psoralen can be toxic to the liver and can cause cataracts. Usually the oral psoralen is restricted to children over ten or so.

Topical PUVA is used if the patches cover less than 20 percent of the body. Oral PUVA is used for more extensive vitiligo (multiple patches totaling more than 20% of the body) or if the skin didn't respond to topical PUVA.

Both treatments require a wait for the psoralen to enter the skin; 2 hours for the oral; 1/2 hour for the topical. Treatments can't be given two days in a row and usually 2-3 treatments a week are given. Patients have to avoid sun for a day and wear 100% UVA/UVB sunglasses for a day as well.

PUVA's mechanism for treating vitiligo: the psoralen in the skin absorbs energy from the UVA light. This energy slows the speed of skin cell multiplication, which is helpful in psoriasis. In vitiligo, the benefits are that the skin's immune response is dampened, T-cells and their cytokines are slowed, and melanocytes increase their distribution of melanin to the keratinocytes.

Side effects of oral psoralen include nausea, vomiting, headache and liver toxicity. Both oral and topical psoralen can result in skin itching, redness, stinging, and/or burning, abnormal hair growth, over tanning, keratitis and cataracts, skin aging/wrinkling and skin cancers.

Burns from treatment are fairly common and not like real sunburn; the burns are from the toxic effects in the skin and take longer to heal. Serious second-degree burns have occurred from errors at the office in timing the UVA and from patients sunbathing right after treatment.

People with hypersensitivity to the sun such as those with lupus or cutaneous porphyrias should avoid PUVA; pregnant women and fertile men and women are counseled to take birth control methods to avoid birth defects during treatment or avoid PUVA.

Narrow Band UVB

While UVB is the cause of sunburn, the wavelengths that cause sunburn do not cover the entire UVB spectrum. Narrow band light therapy takes advantage of this. The range that causes sunburn is generally below 300 nm. Narrow band UVB (nbUVB) lamps produce extremely few waves below 300nm. These few waves around 300nm produced by nbUVB lamps are used in setting treatment times: a little redness that develops the day after treatment and is gone by the following day is often used as a guide for the correct exposure time.

Narrow band UVB provides treatment for vitiligo that is better than PUVA. While it takes just as long – 1-2 years of 3 treatments a week – and half of pigments fade within 2 years, nbUVB almost always provides a more natural matching color whereas fewer than half of PUVA repigmenting match well.

Treatments are less of a burden for the patients: there is no drug, no drug side effects, no need to wear wrap around protective sunglasses after treatments. For some, they can do the treatments at home. For smaller patches, inexpensive nbUVB hand held lamps are available. While expensive, a large panel of nbUVB lights is less expensive than the multiple trips to an office for treatment. (Cost of single 6-foot panel nbUVB lights range from $2000 - $3000 (1232-1848£); full panel lights require a physician's prescription.)

The total body is given nbUVB therapy when generalized vitiligo covers over 15-20% of the body. It's effective on patches that are spreading. Smaller areas of skin are treated with targeted therapy; targeted therapy is moving from nbUVB to excimer lasers described later. Treatment is generally stopped after three months if there's no reaction and after six months if only 25% is repigmented.

It is assumed that nbUVB light stimulates the melanocytes at the boundary of the vitiligo patches and within hair follicles throughout the patches to cause repigmenting. Whole body light therapy may also stabilize existing patches by dampening the immune system.

The major side effect of nbUVB light is from treatments lasting too long and causing burns. Full body treatments also cause tanning of the normal skin, which increases the contrast with the vitiligo areas during treatment.

Excimer lasers and lamps

Excimer laser
The excimer laser began to be used in dermatology in the early 2000s. This equipment delivers a focused, powerful narrow band of UVB pulsed light at 308 nm to a half-inch area. Studies showed the laser to be at least as effective as the nbUVB light at 311nm but took less than half the time for repigmenting to occur. The small focus is useful in treating just the vitiligo patch and has pretty much replaced nbUVB for targeted phototherapy.

As with other phototherapies, the face, scalp and neck have the best results, with variable results for the hands, feet and shins. Segmental vitiligo patches do less well; darker skin has the best outcomes. As with all vitiligo treatments, treatment early in the disease generally provides better outcomes.

Treatments are usually given twice a week, with at least a day in between. Side effects are burning, stinging, and blistering if too much light is given. Generally, practitioners try for a redness of the skin that lasts a day or two. Repigmented areas are fairly stable.

Excimer Lamp

The excimer lamp is a much less expensive form of light therapy that delivers a 308 nm light to the skin. So far studies have shown that the lamp is equivalent to the excimer laser for treating psoriasis, and a few studies have had the same result for vitiligo. A powerful, sealed gas xenon-chloride lamp is the light source. The light source is a steady, less focused beam of light than the pulsed excimer laser. The spot size of the lamps was larger than the lasers when first introduced; manufacturers of both lasers and lamps have been increasing the spot sizes available to reduce treatment times and allow both more efficient treatment and treatment of larger areas.

UVA1

The UVA spectrum of the sun's rays is the one that doesn't cause sunburn. It penetrates deeper into the skin than UVB and causes aging of the skin, wrinkles, and may have a role in some skin cancers.

High strength UVA rays do cause tanning, and quickly. This is what drives the tanning bed industry – they use high power UVA rays and screen out most of the UVB rays. This causes tanning without burning if dosed correctly.

The sun delivers about 5 J/cm^2 and tanning beds about 60 J/cm^2. And the UVA1 lamps now used in dermatology offices have a low/med/hi range of 40/80/130+ J/cm^2.

The UVA1 lamp was invented to research UVA rays on the skin. A lamp was developed that used the longer of the A waves and concentrated the power of them until some biological effect on the skin could be demonstrated and studied.

The UVA1 lamp has been used effectively in atopic dermatitis, scleroderma, cutaneous T-cell lymphoma, and on HIV-1 papules and plaques. Treatment is usually given 5 days a week for 3-4 months. Side effects include over tanning and red, dry, or itching skin. It may activate herpes simplex and may cause skin cancer.

Because of the quick and deep tanning that the UVA1 lamp causes, it seemed like a natural light source for repigmenting vitiligo. Research has also shown UVA to cause T cells to diminish, another target for vitiligo treatments. So far, however, the UVA1 lamp has not been shown to be useful as the single source for vitiligo treatment at the current strengths. Many UVA1 vitiligo research projects are underway.

Red light

Another light source being studied is the low power "cool" helium-neon laser. This laser produces a visible red light at 632.8 nm at a power of 3J/cm^2. In the 1960s, researchers found the light would speed hair regrowth on mice and speed wound healing. A short wave light, it penetrates the skin. It's used for pain relief, wound healing, and removing wrinkles. The light increases collagen production and activates ATP in muscles to release injury.

A few *in vitro* studies have shown the light to induce melanocyte migration and multiplication. A study on patients with segmental vitiligo (which have not shown great responses to other phototherapies) – 60% had marked repigmentation after an average of 17 treatments given 1-2 times a week. Its success with the segmental vitiligo patients has been attributed to the light stimulating sympathetic nerve growth. (Damage to the sympathetic nerves is thought to be a causative factor of segmental vitiligo.)

Red light has no known side effects. As with the excimer laser, a less expensive clinical form to deliver red light treatment has been developed and uses a cluster of LED lights at the same wavelength.

6. Surgical treatments

Surgical techniques are useful in repigmenting small areas of skin that are cosmetically bothersome to patients and which have resisted other treatments. These areas are often the backs of the fingers, around the ankles, shins, knees, elbows, and on the forehead. Each technique attempts to transplant existing melanocytes from pigmented areas of a patient's skin to a vitiligo-affected area.

These treatments can be very effective and long lasting. The downside is cost (most insurance payment is lacking), available technology (transplants occur at larger institutions), infections, and poor color matching with the surrounding skin. Patients who scar easily are not good candidates for any of the surgical treatments.

Surgical methods are only used for patients whose vitiligo is stable – no growth in patches for two years or so is best. It's a good sign if a patient has experienced some spontaneous repigmentation. Patients cannot have had any new Koebner's phenomena – otherwise the trauma of the surgery itself can create more vitiligo patches. If there is any doubt, test treatments are made on a small area.

Mulekarl & Isedeh 92013) each reviewed every surgical article in English with more than three vitiligo patients between 1985 and 2013. Their opinion was that split-thickness grafts and blister grafts were the safest and most effective for medium and small areas. Larger areas treated by the transfer and transplant methods are almost as effective. The transfer/transplant methods are technically feasible to cover very large areas but they thought the pain for the patient and the reported repigmentation rates point to limiting the area covered in any one treatment to about 36 inch^2 (a square 6x6 inches). They concluded that all surgical methods were excellent for focal and segmental vitiligo and thought they should perhaps be considered earlier in treatment.

Several methods have been used to transplant melanocytes to the treated area. They differ in what is taken from the donor site (the area the patient agrees to use skin from) and may differ in the preparation of the vitiligo or treated site.

Whole thickness skin
This is done by punching out small pieces of skin from donor areas, then inserting them into holes punched in the vitiligo site. The recipient holes are smaller to allow a secure fit. The transplanting is usually successful in that the grafts take, but the appearance can give a marbling effect.

Changes in the procedure have included taking "micro" punches (less than 1.5 mm vs 2-3 mm for non-micro punch) and careful control to make the height of the donor piece less than the depth of the vitiligo hole. If the donor piece is higher than the vitiligo hole, the final result is an undesired, uneven 'cobblestone' effect.

Motorized punchers make this procedure able to cover quite a large area at once. The treated area is usually covered with skin adhesive (such as Dermabond) and firm dressing. Care is given that the skin of the treated area does not receive any tension – even to the need to splint to protect skin at or around joints.

The top area blackens and falls off in about two weeks. The pink skin beneath then begins to darken and repigment, going outwards. Topical and/or light therapies are given until the desired pigmentation is reached. The procedure is about 90% successful. Some grafts don't take; some grafts survive but melanocytes don't migrate to untreated skin. More than one treatment may be needed to complete an area.

Split thickness graft – epidermis with a partial layer of dermis
A dermatome (a precise surgical instrument) is used to slice very thin sheets of epidermis/dermis from the donor site. These are left in normal saline for about a week before applying to the prepared vitiligo site.

Dermabrasion or laser is generally used on the vitiligo area; skin is peeled until tiny drops of blood appear. The sheets of epithelium/partial dermis are then placed onto the prepared site.

Pressure and immobilization of the treated area is incredibly important for the graft to adhere to the vitiligo area and become vascularized. The graft has a tendency to shrink so is applied to overlap normal skin. Surgical adhesive and pressure dressings are applied.

The procedure could be painful. Different types of anesthesia are used depending upon how large an area is treated – from general anesthesia, regional block, injecting the edge of treated areas with anesthetic and topical anesthetics.

When the skin has healed, nbUVB is used if needed. Success is in the 80-90% range for this technique. Medium sized areas can be treated and pigmentation is usually good to excellent. The downside of this technique is the "tire patch" look that can occur if the skin color mismatches.

Variations of the split-thickness procedure include:

Cutting the graft into a mesh to cover a wider area and to be more flexible if not being placed over a flat area.

A sandwich technique; pulling back the epidermis, leaving one end still attached, placing the graft, and then putting the epidermis back. This gives a good cover for the healing wound.

Epidermis

Epidermis from the vitiligo area is removed through suction blister, abrasion, freezing or laser. (Some feel using suction blister gives the best cosmetic result.) The epidermis from the donor area is separated from the dermis using suction to raise an epidermal blister from the patient's donor site. The epidermis is cut from the blister and grafted onto the prepared vitiligo site. About a ½ cm is left between grafts, which will fill in. Grafts fall off in about 2 weeks. This method is thought not to be true grafting but a form of melanocyte transfer.

Using solely epidermis gives a good color match. Graft techniques like punch and split thickness that contain dermis are thought to transfer attributes of the donor skin, including color, to the treated area. This procedure takes a long time – 2-3 hours just to form the blisters – and can be painful.

Patients are later treated with topicals and or light therapy to hasten and improve outcomes. This procedure has an 80-90% success with repigmentation averaging about 75%.

Cultured epidermis

Cultured epidermis is a common technique to make sheets of epidermis from small skin sample from the patient. One of the more common uses is for covering large areas of burn patients.

Skin is removed from the donor site and treated to release individual cells, which are spread onto a substrate of irradiated cells. In about three weeks an epithelial film of the patients' cells can be separated from the substrate and placed onto the prepared vitiligo area.

Many methods are used to prepare – i.e. remove the epidermis from – the vitiligo areas. The method used depends upon the dermatologist's preference and experience. Methods include mechanical abrasion, Timedsurgery (brand of programmable electromagnetic waves) and laser.

After two weeks of being bandaged, patients avoid the sun for 3-4 months. Fairly large skin areas can be covered in one session.

Skin cells
In these procedures, a thin slice of the patient's donor skin is shaved, minced and treated with enzymes and acid. The cells are then washed and placed directly on prepared vitiligo skin or just the melanocytes are isolated and cultured to increase the number of available cells for transplant.

The direct application of a cell suspension of melanocytes and keratinocytes is feasible in many places, while the transplant technologies require a more sophisticated lab. These techniques can increase by ten the area that the donor sample can cover.

Needling
Needling has had some success when used in combination with nbUVB or laser light. The borders of vitiligo patches and areas near pigmented hair are pricked multiple times before UV exposure. Pricking goes from the edge to the white area, over and over. The process uses tiny needles, topical anesthetics, and is repeated several times a week and for several months. It has shown some success.

In a variation of this technique, transplant needling, researchers have removed a piece of the patient's skin and divided it into tiny pieces (less than 0.5mm) and implanted these pieces using needling technique.

71

7. Combination treatments

In addition to the growing list of possible individual treatments, clinicians have discovered that combining existing treatments have improved the speed of repigmentation as well as the ability to treat patches that didn't react to any one treatment by itself. A fairly long list of treatments that have been tried can be found in a review by the European Dermatology Forum Consensus (2013). The consensus was that the following have been effective in research studies, but warn that long-term safety of combining two immune suppressors needs studying.

- Phototherapy given for three to four weeks following surgical treatments is effective.
- Potent topical steroids for the first 3 months (taking one week off each month) of phototherapy is effective.
- Topical calcineurin inhibitors tacrolimus (Protopic) and Pimocrolimus (Elidel) have also had positive results with phototherapy.

8. Depigmentation therapies

Depigmentation is the choice for patients with overwhelming vitiligo covering 80% of their bodies. Other patients may choose depigmentation if they have less total body coverage but their disease is progressing and not being helped by other methods. Still others opt to have just their exposed skin depigmented. Generally depigmentation is not pursued for children, with the hope that new treatments now being studied will be effective.

Michael Jackson was among those well-known people who finally chose depigmentation. This is a difficult choice for those with dark skin as it poses cultural and social conflict.

Depigmentation treatments include creams, lasers, chemical peeling, and cryotherapy. Combination treatments are also used.

After successful treatment, patients must avoid sun exposure, use sunscreen and wear protective clothing.

Surprising to many, depigmentation can be as frustrating as repigmenting strategies. Not all the treatments work; even after apparent successful depigmentation, reversals occur.

Topical treatments
All of the topicals irritate the skin to some extent; burns, dermatitis, eczema, brown spots on the whites of the eye may occur with some of them. The chemicals can be absorbed into the body and cause depigmentation in areas not being treated. They also present a potential systemic toxic threat. A slight cancer risk is present for some.

MBEH
A topical cream that is approved for this use in the US is MBEH (monobenzylether of hydroquinone). MBEH kills melanocytes in the skin but not in hair follicles. MBEH was a product in rubber gloves made in the 1930s that caused vitiligo-like patches of the hands as well as areas thought to be caused by the systemic spread of the chemical. When the gloves stopped being used, the workers' hands recovered their pigment

The cream is sometimes sold commercially; more often a compounding pharmacy is needed to provide strengths up to 40%. The more common strength is 20%. After skin testing for a period to test for allergic reaction on normal skin, the cream is applied 1-2 times a day until depigmentation occurs – which may be a few months to as long as two years. Use of the cream near the eyes is not recommended. Fading of the skin is usually apparent in 1-3 months. The darker the skin the longer it takes.

Side effects of treatment include dermatitis and brown spots on the whites of the eye. Repigmentation can occur – thought to be from exposing hair follicles in the affected area to sunlight.

Patients are warned not to have MBEH-treated skin come in contact with other person's skin.

Various authors cite 60-90% success rates with MBEH. The depigmented color is the same flat white of a vitiligo patch. If the white patch is whiter than the patients' vitiligo patch, patients may tint their skin by taking oral beta-carotene.

Given the excitement over developing therapies, patients are warned that the depigmentation is generally permanent and would lessen the chance of repigmentation at a later date.

MBEH + Tretinoin
Tretinoin (all trans retinoic acid or ATRA) is used for treatment of acne. It has been found to enhance melanocyte death and when used with MBEH shortens treatment time. The concentration is usually 0.025-0.1%. Side effects include hyperpigmentation and skin irritation. Milder forms of retinoid have been proposed.

4MP
Monomethyl ether of hydroquinone (4MP) is a substance similar to MBEH. One brand, Mcquinol, is generally used as a 20% concentration in a cream and applied twice a day. It is easier on the skin than MBEH and can be combined with Tretinoin. It takes longer to depigment an area but is more easily tolerated. 4MP is less expensive than MBEH but is not available in the required high concentration in the US.

(4MP is an ingredient in Solange, a product available in the US recommended for fading solar lentigines – liver spots. The 4MP is in a concentration of 2% solution combined with Tretinoin 0.01% in alcohol.)

Phenol
Phenol in a high (88%) concentration is commonly used for skin peeling. It has been used for both depigmenting and pigmenting in vitiligo.

When applied to the skin it causes it to coagulate and peel off. The coagulated skin keeps the phenol from penetrating too deeply. The procedure requires the skin to be carefully cleaned, then the phenol is dabbed on and the skin turns white. The patient feels a sharp burn, then it lessens. Then there is some pain as the area heals over for two weeks or so. Antibiotic/steroid preparations are applied. Antivirals are used if the patient has had herpes simplex.

The process is repeated again in about 40-60 days. When used on the face and neck, about 20% of the area can be treated at once. Larger areas cannot be treated all at once because some of the phenol enters the blood stream and is extremely toxic to the liver.

The benefit of this procedure is that it is fairly quick to perform and inexpensive. Results are almost immediate. Repigmenting may occur with sun exposure. Scarring and unwanted skin color may occur. Some patients have cardiovascular problems several hours after the procedure.

When used in a repigmenting process, the skin peel is followed by PUVA or other treatment. It has been reported to be more successful in treating stable vitiligo than standard treatments alone.

Cryotherapy
Cryotherapy is an inexpensive depigmenting therapy but, because of the scarring risk, should only be used by experienced dermatologists. Some will only treat very small areas while others will treat the same amount of skin as for phenol. Cryotherapy is often used to treat areas that haven't reacted to MBEH.

Usually the skin is frozen using probes cooled with liquid nitrogen or CO_2 cryogun for 10-30 seconds depending upon the technology used. The freezing causes ice crystals to form inside the melanocytes and kill them. There is pain, blistering, and extreme redness and oozing wounds, which can be alarming.

When the skin recovers in four to six weeks, the procedure is repeated one or two more times. While painful and requiring careful care of the healing skin for several months, the results are usually fairly stable. Success has been reported with one cryotherapy session followed by topical 4-HP.

Lasers

Various Q switch lasers (532-1064nm) have been used to depigment the remaining skin of vitiligo patients. The best results have been with patients with active disease, especially those who experience Koebner's phenomena – whose skin reacts to trauma with new depigmentation. (About a third of patients with generalized vitiligo experience Koebner's.) The Q switch lasers emit powerful pulses of light and are used to remove freckles, tattoos, and other skin blemishes. Their various wavelengths are designed for different colors and skin penetration. For this use in vitiligo, melanocytes absorb the energy of the laser and die. The procedure hurts and topical anesthetics may be used. The procedure itself is fairly quick and large areas can be treated. Patients see outcomes within a few weeks. Usually a spot is tested first to see if the laser will be effective. If the spot is not depigmented, further laser treatment is not attempted.

After treatment, the skin turns red and blisters appear. During the healing process, the area is usually kept moist for about a week to prevent scarring. Each dermatologist will have a different strategy to do this. Then the area is allowed to dry.

Several sessions may be required. Repigmentation does occur, especially among patients with stable vitiligo. Reports of improved results from having the patient tan before treatment to activate the melanocytes have been made.

Topical MBEH and 4-MP used during treatment have been reported to improve results and decrease the number of laser treatments needed. Research continues on the lasers and topical therapies best for this procedure.

Chapter 7: Other Remedies

Because there is no one treatment for vitiligo that always works, works quickly and inexpensively, and has no side effect – there have been hundreds of compounds put forth as treatments. Compounds in this section are those mentioned frequently in literature and in patient reports as either treatments or as helpful adjuncts to treatment. Some have shown promise and are being studied.

Patients who have tried one or two medical treatments that haven't worked are apt to try anything. If they do not have a medical professional to guide them through this maze, I urge them to at least consult monitored websites and social networking sites to assure their safety. Those offered by the major vitiligo support organizations and many of the Facebook and similar groups can help.

1. Vitamins

Healthy skin depends upon a healthy body. Specific vitamins and other substances mentioned in literature as important for healthy skin are Vitamins A,B,C,D, E and K and silica, zinc, DMAE (dimethylaminoethanol), coenzyme Q10, and omega 3 fatty acids.

Not surprising, items on the "healthy skin" list are also found in descriptions of vitiligo "diets" as well as topical products thought to help. Below are some facts about each one as well as their possible role in vitiligo.

Vitamin A

Vitamin A, or retinol, is a fat-soluble substance that can be toxic if taken to excess. Dietary sources include livers, milk, butter, and some cheeses; carrots, broccoli, sweet potatoes, kale and peas

Role in the skin: Vitamin A is a strong antioxidant. Vitamin A also helps regulate cell growth and epithelial integrity and modulates the immune response.

Shortage in vitiligo? No specific shortage has been reported in vitiligo patients, although epithelial deficiency has been theorized. Vitamin A deficiency is rare in developed countries.

Use in vitiligo: No dietary or supplement of Vitamin A beyond that recommended for anyone.

As retinol is used in creams to fade dark skin spots, topical vitamin A is not recommended.

Vitamin B 12 & Folate (B9)

Both vitamin Bs are water soluble. Vitamin B12 is found in animal products such as meat, shellfish, milk, cheese and eggs. Folate is found in leafy greens, eggs, liver, citrus, corn, broccoli, and many fortified foods. Folic acid is the manufactured supplement for folate.

These vitamins are essential for making DNA and regulate nervous systems, circulatory components, and energy. Folic acid is damaged by heat and stomach acid so it added to bread and cereals. Vitamin B12 shortage happens more commonly in adults, as it requires good stomach acid to absorb from food. The B vitamins are involved in the metabolism of every cell of the human body, especially affecting DNA synthesis and regulation, but also fatty acid synthesis and energy production

Role in the skin: Homocysteine is an amino acid found in blood plasma. Its levels are controlled by B12 and folate. Patients with deficiencies of these vitamins often have high homocysteine levels, narrowed arteries, and other cardiovascular problems thought to result from oxidative stress. The same occurs in skin, with high levels of hydrogen peroxide, which damages or kills melanocytes. High homocysteine levels can also cause a reduction in methioline needed for melanin production.

Shortage in vitiligo? Yes. Low levels of B12 and folic acid in the blood have been found in a large number of vitiligo patients.

Use in vitiligo: Oral supplements coupled with sun or nbUVB have been effective in repigmenting vitiligo patches, especially in children.

Patients are warned not to experiment with B12 and Folic acid supplements without a physician's advice. Too much folic acid coupled with low B12 can cause neurological damage.

Vitamin C

Most animals can make their own Vitamin C, but humans cannot. It is found in many fruits & vegetables, seafood, and animal meats – especially liver, and added to many food products. Vitamin C is an antioxidant and reduces body damage from free radicals.

Role in the skin: Vitamin C has a role in collagen synthesis, skin repair, and the strength and firmness of skin. Through its antioxidant properties it can reduce effects of oxidative stress. In addition, Vitamin C is thought to have a role in regenerating oxidized vitamin E, another important antioxidant.

Shortage in vitiligo? There have been some reports of low levels of vitamin C in a few Vitiligo patients, but it occurs much less frequently than in B12 and folate.

Use in vitiligo: One study reported from the University of Alabama that Vitamin C added to a B12/folate supplement increased repigmentation (Montes, 1992). Vitamin C is often recommended as part of multivitamins for vitiligo. Some patients report Vitamin C as causing their patches to spread; guesses as to causes have included food allergy.

Vitamin D

Vitamin D is a fat-soluble substance. Vitamin D is found in fish, eggs, liver and fortified milk and cereal. The body can make Vitamin D from cholesterol and the sun. The vitamin has a role in the body's absorption of calcium and other compounds from the gut and in regulating calcium in the bones. Vitamin D has some antioxidant properties and supports the immune system.

Vitamin D is broken down in the liver and kidney to calcitriol, the active form of the vitamin.

Fish & shellfish, eggs, liver, and mushrooms are among the few natural food sources of Vitamin D; orange juice and milk are among the products commonly fortified with it.

Role in the skin: Studies have demonstrated Vitamin D receptors on all skin cells as well as T-cells and B-cells – pointing towards a role in the immune system.

Shortage in vitiligo? As many patients are told to avoid sunlight, many naturally have low vitamin D levels. Many physicians now tell their patients to have up to 15 minutes of natural sunlight every day before putting on sunscreen.

What interests researchers about vitiligo and Vitamin D is the relationship with autoimmune diseases. When vitamin D levels were measured in a group of vitiligo patients, for example, low levels of D were associated with a marked increase in the number of patients who also had another autoimmune disease. The

Vitamin D levels were not associated with the severity of the vitiligo.

Use in vitiligo: Topical vitamin D analogues (manufactured vitamin similar in structure to D) have been developed and tried as topical treatment for vitiligo; these include calcitriol and paricalcitol. The action hoped for has been stimulation of melanocytes. There are no serious side effects – dry skin, burning, stinging. They've had limited success when used alone but have added a positive effect when used with topical steroids and/or nbUVB.

Vitamin E

Vitamin E is soluble in fat and is a well-known antioxidant. It regulates some enzyme and neurological functions and mediates gene expression. It's found in a wide variety of vegetables, oils, meat, eggs, poultry, and cereals.

Role in the skin: Vitamin E protects skin against cancer and wrinkles

Shortage in vitiligo? Low vitamin E has been reported in the skin of some vitiligo patients.

Use in vitiligo: Oral vitamin E is used in vitiligo for its antioxidant properties. Used alone, as an oral supplement, it has weak repigmenting properties. It is often used in combination with other therapies. It's one of those substances that seems hopeful as a treatment but has not yet been proven terribly effective.

2. L-Phenylalanine

L-Phenylalanine is an essential amino acid found in meat, eggs, fish, cheese, some nuts, soy, and the artificial sweetener, Aspartame. L-phenylalanine is important in protein synthesis.

Role in the skin: L-Phenylalanine is metabolized to tyrosine, a compound essential in melanin production.

Shortage in vitiligo? None reported.

Role in vitiligo? One study showed repigmentation with oral supplements. Oral supplement with topical treatment at the same time with sun or UVA or nbUVB has showed greater repigmentation. It is thought that UV light speeds conversion of phenylalanine to tyrosine.

As with many treatments being tried, this one is said to warrant further study.

Many concoctions of vitamins, minerals, etc. sold as a vitiligo supplement contain L-Phenylalanine. Patients should not take these without consulting a specialist. High doses of phenylalanine cause nerve damage and lower doses can trigger allergies, cause nausea, anxiety, insomnia, and interfere with high blood pressure. In addition, patients with PKU should not take this compound.

3. Coenzyme Q10

Coenzyme Q10 is a compound much like a vitamin – except it is produced in the body (vitamins aren't). It's an intracellular antioxidant in one of its reduced forms and helps enzymes work in energy production. It's found in almost every cell – in the membrane of those cells with nuclei. While it's found in the body, it is also in several foods such as organ meats, sardines, some nuts, and soy.

Role in the skin: Coenzyme Q10 decreases with age and the lack of it in the skin is thought to be one of the causes of wrinkles. Its most important role is the generation of energy within cells; when it's in a reduced state (hydroquonone) it can swap its electrons to capture free radicals and prevent cell damage.

Shortage in vitiligo? Low concentration of Coenzyme Q10 has been reported in active vitiligo skin in concert with low Vitamin E.

Use in vitiligo: Coenzyme Q10 has been studied in vitiligo. In one study, which only ran eight weeks, oral Q10 produced some pigmentation. It also reduced the amount of serum MDA (melonialdehyde), a marker for oxidative stress.

Coenzyme Q10 is often recommended for vitiligo patients along with other vitamins, minerals, and antioxidants. It can cause insomnia and a drop in blood sugar. At high doses it can cause skin rashes and GI symptoms.

Topical coenzyme Q10 has been reported to trigger vitiligo – perhaps not surprising as the reduced form of Q10, hydroquonone, is used in skin creams to erase age spots and other dark skin blemishes.

4. Gingko biloba

The gingko tree is native to China. It is said to be a relic, a fossil – as it has no living tree relatives. The leaves, fruit and seeds of the tree have been used for food and medicines for millennia. The seeds contain a toxin but extracts from the leaf are widely used today.

The plant extracts have antioxidant and anti-inflammatory properties. Extracts have been shown to increase blood flow.

Use in vitiligo: Oral gingko has been successful in two small clinical trials: it stopped the progression of the spread of vitiligo and caused some repigmentation. This is without any light therapy or other treatment. Which properties of the leaf are responsible is still being studied. It is thought to be gingko's ability to dampen autoimmune response and oxidative stress associated with vitiligo. Gingko may also benefit the skin by increasing circulation to clear toxins more effectively.

Gingko is a blood thinner so should not be used with other OTC or prescribed blood thinners without a physician's knowledge. It also interacts with a number of prescription drugs. By itself, and within dosages used so far, it has few side effects beyond possible GI disturbances and skin allergies.

5. Minerals

Zinc, silica, and other minerals have been reported to cause repigmentation but have not been studied.

6. The sun

As noted earlier in the book, the earliest treatments for vitiligo were discovered centuries ago by persons eating or applying sun sensitizing plants, seeds – or extracts of them – on their vitiligo areas and then going into the sun. Through experimentation, they discovered what worked. including how much sun to apply. PUVA treatment is the offshoot of this ancient research.

People throughout the world still use their own concoctions using seeds or leafs from health food stores and trade recipes on the internet. I can only urge caution for anyone with vitiligo to "go it alone". There are so many products out there which are either useless, can make vitiligo worse, or have other adverse health effects.

In formal medicine, some physicians prescribe topical steroids or other melanin sensitizing compounds for their patients to use with careful exposure to the sun. One medication, PUVA-Sol, is intended for this use. Care must be used in any of these instances as serious sunburns can occur, which can trigger vitiligo spread rather than repigmentation.

The use of nbUVB with these medications or herbs would be safer, as it avoids most of the burning UVB rays from the sun. They are also more powerful and speed repigmenting. There are both 308nm and 311nm lights available from handheld lamps for focal patches to large panels. Most online sellers do not require a physician's prescription but coach that one would be helpful in getting insurance reimbursement for one. As with the use of any vitamin or natural product, a physician who treats vitiligo should advise the selection of the lamp and compounds used with it.

7. Michael Dawson

Michael Dawson's website is unavoidable to anyone researching vitiligo. Any combination of vitiligo and another search word will land you on his site. I mention this because to leave the site you have to beg. His treatment, according to online patient reports, consists of a reasonable combination of B12, B complex, folic acid, vitamin E, gingko, and moisturize skin with coconut oil. (I have not read his book.)

8. Melagenia Plus

Melagenia Plus is an alcohol lipoprotein extraction from human placentas with added calcium. It's sold in Cuba and on the Internet and advertises that it can cure vitiligo 86% of the time and has no side effects. In some ads it says it transplants melanocytes. One used to have to go to Cuba for diagnosis and treatment but now it's available online for $130 for 235 ml/8 oz. (80£). The instructions are to rub it into the skin once a day and to avoid the sun. Repigmentation is not guaranteed and if it works it could take months or years.

Nordlund & Halder (1990) reviewed published data in an article for Dermatologica and noted that "The biochemistry, assays for biological activity and the pharmacology studies as reported do not stand up to rigorous and acceptable scientific standards."

They did not rule the product as not useful but hoped that it could be studied in depth as any purported treatment for vitiligo.

A study published by Majid in 2010 compared UVB and UVB plus melagenia and reported that the placental drug had no significant effect on vitiligo repigmentmentation.

9. Ayurvedic Treatments

Ayurvedic Medicine is based upon an ancient system in India. There were over 1200 medicinal plants in the Ayurvedic formulary, which was trimmed to the 200 most useful plants in the 1950s. The treatment most often prescribed for vitiligo is Bakuchi, made from leaves of the Psoralea corylifolia plant. This is our old friend psoralen. This is usually given in tablet form with or without phototherapy. Liver toxicity has been reported, probably because Bakuchi is sometimes prescribed to be taken every day, while in PUVA treatment, oral or topical psoralen is given just before UVA treatment two or three times a week and at lower doses.

Another plant, Picrorhiza kurra, is prescribed to enhance the effects of Bakuchi as a psorolen enhancer. This compound can act to stimulate the immune system and be counterproductive in vitiligo.

Many preparations of Ayurvedic treatments are combinations of several plants and should be viewed with caution. Heavy metals (arsenic and mercury) and other potentially toxic materials may be included.

10. Novitil

Novitil is a commercial natural therapy that is combined with a therapeutic light source. Many have reported positive results when using it as directed. Novitil does not require a prescription. Users are told to apply the gel to vitiligo areas twice a day, and then use the sun, infrared light, or cautiously use a UVB/UVA tanning bed. They are to keep the gel in place for two hours each time.

Novitil contains distilled water, lipoproteins, polypeptides, Aloe barbadensis, carboxymethylcellulose, camphor, menthol and oligoelements and kathon. According to Yoon et al. (2011), only aloe barbadensis may have anti-inflammatory activity in vitiligo, but other ingredients listed do not have proven anti-vitiligo effects.

11. Pseudocatalase

Catalase is an antioxidant enzyme found in healthy skin but in low levels in the skin of vitiligo patients. In the skin, catalase breaks down hydrogen peroxide (a common byproduct of metabolism) into water and oxygen, protecting melanocytes. It's sensible to try to see if replacing the enzyme would help in vitiligo treatment.

Dr. Karin Schallreuter developed a pseudocatalase cream, PC-KUS, in Germany and has reported great success in repigmenting vitiligo lesions: she reports that greater than 60% of patients have positive outcomes; of those with positive outcomes –lesions are repigmented by 95%. The cream is applied over the body twice a day, and used with sunlight or nbUVB twice a week. Schallreuter's group also ran successful experiments with patients first submerging in the Dead Sea, said to have some components of catalase, before the PC-KUS treatment. Schallreuter has also measured hydrogen peroxide before and after PC-KUS treatment and shown a significant decrease.

So far, PC-KUS is available only through Schallreuter's group in Germany and England; the formula is patented. It is now being put forward as a cure for gray hair.

A reverse-engineered product is available from some US and Canadian compounding pharmacies which is called pseudocatalase or PCAT, but this formula has not been found effective in studies.

PCAT has been reported to cause acne and ingrown hairs and is reported to be ineffective for patients with phenylalanine deficiency.

12. Vitiligo Herb™ and Anti-Vitiligo™

These products and others like them contain psorolen-like compounds, antioxidants, and anti-inflammatory substances. Users need to be cautious in their use with sun or other forms of phototherapy.

13. Homeopathic Compounds

No compounds from homeopathic medicine have been found useful for vitiligo.

14. Additional Compounds

Bee venom (injected into lesions), pepper extracts, minocycline.

15. Compounds to Avoid

Generally, a healthy diet is recommended. Patients should avoid prepared foods with long lists of additives. There are just a few foods to be cautious of, but most important is for each vitiligo patient to be aware of any food eaten right before a flare-up.

- Fish from areas with heavy metals or toxins such as dioxin and mercury should be avoided. If allergic or sensitive to nickel, foods containing this metal should be avoided:

- Picrorhiza: activates the immune system, not recommended for vitiligo.
- Blueberries and pears contain natural depigmenting agents.
- Vitamin C and turmeric cause depigmenting in some patients. (But most patients can eat food with vitamin C and use it in supplements.)
- Echinacea stimulates the immune system and should be avoided as well as similar plant extracts including goldenseal, astragalus, and spirulina.
- Ginseng can aggravate vitiligo except in tiny amounts.
- Paraphenylene Diamine (PDPA) in hair dyes.
- Imiquimod treatment for other skin conditions can cause vitiligo to flare up.
- Fragrances in many products can be harmful for vitiligo patients; use of fragrance free products is recommended.
- Mouthwashes and toothpastes with thimerosal.
- Musk or cinnamic aldehyde in cosmetics (and nanoparticles for now).
- Phenols in hair dyes.

Chapter 8: Treatment Guidelines

In recent years, organizations, physicians, researchers and others have worked to add clarity in treatment of vitiligo for the practicing physician. Summaries of two of the guidelines follow.

1. Anbar et al.

One proposed system for patient flow was published by Anbar et al. (2014) – it is a good place to start and is summarized here. They proposed that:

Active disease is first stabilized with topical or systemic medication

Once stable, group patients by percent body surface area (BSA) covered with lesions. (For reference see Appendix B which contains common rules of thumb for estimating body surface areas of adults and children.)

If greater than 75% of BSA is affected, present depigmentation option. If patient doesn't want, or can't afford treatment, provide information about camouflage. Also, some patients will want camouflage during treatment.

If less than 75% of **BSA** is affected, the treatment approach depends upon whether the hair over the vitiligo lesion has changed, i.e. profuse dark hairs vs. hairs scanty or turned white

If less than 75% of BSA is affected with profuse dark hair:

- Small lesions: target phototherapy, excimer laser, topical medications. If treatment fails, consider surgery.

- Large lesion or multiple small ones: phototherapy, topical medication.
- If treatment fails and less than 20% of surface area is affected, consider surgery.
- If treatment fails and more than 20% surface area is affected, offer camouflage.

If less than 75% BSA is affected, and hair is scanty or white:

- For patches less than 1 cm^2: target phototherapy, excimer laser, or topical medication. If treatment fails, consider surgery.
- For patches greater than 1 cm^2: consider surgery. If surgery fails four times, offer camouflage.

(1 cm^2 is very small: a letter key on standard computer keyboard is 1.69 cm^2)

Why is the type of hair over the vitiligo area important in treatment?

An important source of melanocytes is found in the hair follicle; also melanocyte stem cells are located there. Dark hair over the skin means these melanocytes are still alive. Various treatments stimulate the melanocytes to move to the skin surface and repigment the skin, first around the follicle, then moving outwards. This pattern is also seen in cases of spontaneous regression of vitiligo.

It is especially important to provide early treatment to stop active disease among segmental vitiligo patients. These patients are prone to developing white hairs over the lesions and the opportunity to use follicular melanocytes is critical in their care.

In areas without hair (mucous membranes, palms and soles) any melanocytes for repigmenting have to come from the margins of the vitiligo lesion or through surgical procedures.

Why is the size of the vitiligo area important in treatment?

For lesions without hair, or if the hair is scantier than the surrounding normal skin, or if the hair is white, there are not enough "live" melanocytes from hair follicles. Any melanocytes to repigment have to come from the margin of the vitiligo lesion. Melanocytes can be stimulated to migrate, but the maximum distance they travel is 2-3 mm. Therefore, only small patches can be expected to benefit from medical treatments.

In addition, patients with large lesions or with many small ones are more apt to benefit from whole body phototherapy than trying to target each lesion.

What is considered treatment failure?

Medical options: if no response after 3 months or if unsatisfactory response after 6 months.

Surgical options: if four attempts provide unsatisfactory response

What kind of camouflage do they recommend?

Any temporary camouflage. The medical tattooing can lead to additional lesions through Koebner response; some patients have allergic reactions; many patients have poor color matching; and the color fades.

2. Vitiligo European Task Force (VETF)

The VETF and related European dermatological societies have published several guidelines of the treatments available for vitiligo. The latest was published in 2013 (Taieb, 2013). They divide patients by whether the vitiligo pattern is segmental (SV) or not (NSV). SV occurs early in life, progresses quickly, but generally stabilizes in a few years. SV is thought to have a different etiology from SNV. It is especially important to stabilize SV as soon as possible.

The VETF Guidelines (numbers indicate the order of treatments to try):

For all patients

1. Support and counsel. Access to camouflage instruction.

SV or limited NSV (less than 2-3% BSA)

1. Avoid triggers. Apply topical steroids or calcineurin inhibitors
2. Local phototherapy especially using excimer laser or lamp
3. Surgery

NSV with more than 2-3% BSA affected

1. Avoid triggers. NbUVB for 3 to 9 months in combination with systemic or topical therapy
2. Systemic steroids for 3 to 4 months, minipulse
3. Graft areas of cosmetic importance when stable
4. If vitiligo lesions are greater than 50%, depigment. Areas determined with patient. Using either 4-methoxyphenol or hydroquinone monobenzl ether. Use the depigmenting agents alone or with Q-switched ruby laser.

Special considerations:

- Anti-inflammatory agents are probably helpful to curb inflammation. Agents include methotrexate.
- If melanocyte survival is a concern, growth factor supplements may be helpful. These include MSH (melanocyte stimulating hormone) analogues.
- New repigmenting agents include Helium-Neon laser and Prostaglandin E2. These were mentioned but not evaluated by the task force.

VETF additional comments on specific treatments:

Topical corticosteroids (TCS)

- Excluding the face, can be used daily for 3 months. Better if used 15 days a month for 6 months.
- For children, or if large areas involved, use the strongest TCS with fewest side effects, such as mometasone furoate.

Topical Calcineurin inhibitors (TCI)

For head, neck, thin skin, active vitiligo. Twice a day for 6 months; daily, moderate sun. If effective can be used up to 12 months.

Phototherapy

- NbUVB. Use total body therapy if 15-20% or more BSA is affected.
- Use targeted phototherapy for small, recent lesions and for children.
- No consensus about length of therapy. Many hold to stopping if no repigmentation after 3 months or if unsatisfactory repigmentation after 6 months. If pigmentation is still occurring, can treat up to two years.

Combination therapies

- TCS + phototherapy. Useful on difficult to treat areas such as the shins etc. Daily potent TCS or TCS for three weeks out of four, for 3 months.
- TCI + phototherapy. Appears useful. Long-term cancer risk needs study.
- Vitamin D + phototherapy. Not recommended.
- Oral antioxidants + phototherapy. Needs study.
- Surgery + phototherapy. Improves repigmentation when used for 3-4 weeks following surgery.

Oral Minipulse (OMP) corticosteroids

- OMP not useful for repigmentation.
- Used to stop progression of active vitiligo. Often low daily oral dexamethasone is used for 3 to 6 months. Relapse is common, especially in younger children.

Surgery

- Primarily used in SV and local forms of vitiligo.
- If used for NSV patients, care must be taken to avoid Koebner phenomenon and patients warned of relapse in general.

Camouflage

- Self-tanning. Good choice. Seawater fades but otherwise stable color for 3-5 days.
- Creams with stabilizers. Good color match. Can be stable for a day. Care must be taken to clean skin carefully to avoid sparking Koebner's.
- Tattooing. May be suitable for lips (especially skin types V and VI) and nipples. Iffy for other areas.

Mental Health

- Evaluate patients to see if formal support needed, although no specific treatment has been shown to be particularly effective.
- Patients need to talk about the impact of vitiligo on their lives.
- For teenagers and those with dark skins, community interventions may be needed.

Chapter 9: Research

Many dermatologists are criticized for not being interested in treating vitiligo patients. Look at it from a clinician's point of view for a moment. There have been hundreds of proposed treatments over the years yet none of them cure vitiligo, none of them are effective for all patients, and the long-term safety of those treatments that are effective for some patients is still unknown. Furthermore, many of the reports of vitiligo treatments are clinical reports of a single treatment for one or just a few patients.

In 2011 a group of patients, healthcare professionals and researchers were surveyed for own research priorities in an effort by the James Lind Alliance (JLA) Vitiligo Priority Setting Partnership in the UK. (V. Eleftheriadou et al., 2011)

The 461 participants offered 660 of their top priorities, then whittled them down to their top ten. Looking at them, you can see the issues are extremely basic treatment issues.

- Are systemic immunosuppresants effective?
- Are psychological interventions helpful?
- Which is best: light therapy or calcineurin inhibitors?
- Is UVB therapy combined with topical monotherapies effective?
- Does gene therapy have a role in treatment?
- Are hormones or hormone-related substances such as melanocyte-stimulating hormone analogues and afamelanotide effective?
- Which is better: topical calcineurin inhibitors or corticosteroids?
- Which is better: topical corticosteroids or light therapy?
- Should psychological aid be added to camouflage?

- How effective is pseudocatalase cream plus brief nbUVB

They were also interested to see studies of black pepper (piperine) and stem cell therapy.

There have been numerous shortcomings identified with much of vitiligo clinical research that has been done to guide treatment. In clinical research, the preferred way to test a treatment's efficacy is by randomized controlled trials (RCTs). If a new treatment is being studied, in an RCT some patients are randomly assigned to the new treatment while other patients may be assigned to a current treatment, a placebo, or both. The results are compared using standard statistical methods.

The Cochrane Collaboration is a not-for-profit organization of experts in 120 different countries, which evaluates published medical studies for their validity and suggest changes for future research. They reviewed 218 vitiligo studies and found only 57 that were RTCs. Their 2011 report of vitiligo interventions concluded there was "some evidence" to support existing treatments but the studies couldn't be compared as they used different designs and outcome measures and failed to report on the quality of life of the patients. (Gonzalez, 2011) The report concluded that high quality RCTs were needed, which covered the permanence of repigmentation and assessed the quality of life of the patients. They noted that the long-term permanence of any repigmentation needs to be studied and reported – at least for a year after treatment and ideally at least two years.

In terms of treatment effectiveness, Cochrane thought there was:

- Moderate evidence for topical corticosteroids, but long term treatment wasn't viable because of side effects
- Topical, non-steroidal calcineurin inhibitors were promising, especially when combined with light therapy
- Excimer light may be the best source for phototherapy

- Suction blisters have side effect of new vitiligo at the donor sites

Cochrane was critical of studies that didn't report the age of the patients, skin color, stage of the disease, size of vitiligo lesions, duration of the disease, site of vitiligo patches, and standard verifiable method to measure repigmentation.

In a follow-up review, 33 new studies were added. There was still no long-term follow-up; none measured the spread of lesions; and few mentioned the quality of life. There was greater detail on side effects of treatment but researchers still had their own styles of measuring repigmentation.

In addition to the treatments outlined below, studies include a 10-year follow-up of acrofacial vitiligo patients to see if the description is apt or if patients showed additional vitiligo lesions and a study of hearing in vitiligo patients.

1. Recent studies of potential treatments include:

Implanted afamelanotide (Scenesse®) used with nbUVB.

Afamelanotide, marketed as Scenesse®, mimics a natural hormone that stimulates melanocytes to produce melanin. The natural hormone (alpha-melanocyte stimulating hormone, α-MSH) is very short lived but the manufactured compound is not. Afamelanotide was developed as a drug that could tan without sun thus protecting skin from harmful rays. Afamelanotide specifically acts upon melanocytes to make more eumelanin, the darker black/brown pigment, than pheomelanin, a red/yellow pigment.

Scenesse, marketed by Clinuvel, has already been tested in several clinical trials for skin conditions including some for vitiligo. In the vitiligo trials so far, patients were started with a month of nbUVB treatment, then injected with a 16 mg dissolvable pellet the size of a grain of rice that contained the Scenesse (Grimes, 2013). The Scenesse was injected four times, each a month apart. The trial ended with another month of nbUVB. The control group received nbUVB alone for six months. So far, the results have been encouraging. Patients with skin types III to VI were included in the studies, and those with types IV to VI did the best. In the Phase IIa study, patients getting the Scenesse began showing pigmentation sooner than controls (43rd day vs. 68 days) and were been reported to have more complete and deeper pigmentation.

There were a few GI upsets recorded and some instances of hyperpigmentation. Of the 55 patients in the Stage 11a trial, 13 patients left before finishing – 5 because of over-darkening of normal skin and 8 because of the time demands of the study. A measurement of the changes in the quality of life were attempted and showed no difference. Additional trials are ongoing. Long-term stability of the repigmented lesions is being studied and randomized control studies are planned.

Photocil®

Photocil is an over-the-counter cream produced by Applied Biology. When applied to vitiligo lesions, the cream is said to allow only the nbUVB rays through, preventing more damaging rays from entering. The UVB rays allowed by Photocil peak at 308nm, the same as electric nbUVB lamps. Photocil has been proposed as either a stand-alone treatment, which can mimic nbUVB treatment using natural sunlight for the light source, or in conjunction with other topical or surgical treatments.

The active ingredient in Photocil is dimethicone, silicone oil. The cream is a 1% preparation of dimethicone and includes other skin softening ingredients. Dimethicone is a common ingredient in skin preparations, including Johnson's Baby Cream.

A pilot study showed repigmentation in an 11-week trial in which Photocil was better than placebo (Goren, 2014). All Photocil patients were reported to have repigmentation rates ranging from 30%-70%.

Physicians Institute, Tucson, Arizona, is conducting a clinical study using Photocil alone with sunshine.

Simvastatin

Simvastatin is a drug commonly used to lower cholesterol. Its potential for use as a vitiligo treatment came from a published case report in 2004 of a man with vitiligo and cardiac problems. He noticed his vitiligo patches were much less when he was prescribed simvastatin.

Simvastatin's effect in vitiligo is presumed to be through its anti-inflammatory and antioxidant properties. It is being studied at the University of Massachusetts using an oral dose of 40 mg per day for a month followed by 80 mg per day for five months. The outcome will include VASI scores for the sentinel patch and chemical studies involving cytokines. (Harris, 2011)

Intralesional corticosteroids

Injecting corticosteroids directly into the vitiligo lesions was tried years ago and has lately received new interest. There has been a recent report of success with injecting triamcinolone acetonide, a corticosteroid, into vitiligo lesions. Injections were given every four to five weeks to 9 patients. Injections, given 4-6 weeks apart, provided 80-90% repigmentation within an average of 4 months. Longest treatment was for 7 months.

A formal study of intralesional injections of this drug is ongoing at the University of British Columbia. (Aljasser, 2013)

Neovir

Neovir is a cancer drug manufactured by Pharmsyntez in Russia. The drug is an interferon enhancer and in Russia is an inexpensive over-the-counter medication. In a pilot study announced in 2013, intramuscular injection of Neovir for 60 nonsegmental vitiligo patients stopped active progression for 73% and significant repigmentation in four when followed for 12 months after the injections. (Korobko, 2014)

ACH24

This is named ACH24 for clinical trials proposed by the manufacturer Aché Laboratories of Brazil. The compound is an extract of stachytarpheta cayensensis, a flowering plant of the verbena family. Parts of the plant and flowers are important in Brazil's folk medicine and have anti-inflammatory properties. The study may not have started yet. (Ache, 2011)

Piperine

Western interest in piperine began with a phone call more than 20 years ago from the UK Vitiligo Society to King's College London for information about a mixture of Chinese herbs for vitiligo. Amala Soumyanath, one of the pharmacists there, was a specialist in natural medicines and made a list of ingredients of all the mixtures for vitiligo mentioned in Ayurvedic and Chinese medicine (OHSU, 2013). They tested 30 compounds on cultured mouse melanocytes. One, a water based extract of black pepper, stimulated melanocyte growth and also stimulates dendrite formation. (Dendrites are the "fingers" that sprout from melanocytes to deliver melanin to keratinocytes.)

Several formulations of piperine have been studied *in vitro* using animal and human melanocytes and in animal vitiligo models. Pigmentation occurred with topical piperine in the animals.

Piperine has also been shown to inhibit cell-cultured melanoma cells.

It's been discovered that UV interferes with piperine so any phototherapy, including sunshine, would have to alternate with application of the piperine. Research of the safety of the product continues.

A patent for a piperine compound and its use in vitiligo is now owned by Oregon Health and Science University where Soumyanath now works. AdPharma is licensed to develop it. Human trials have not begun.

Note: Several people have made their own extracts from black pepper or have used pepper oil from health food stores. When asked if this was safe, Soumyanath responded in 2013, "Although piperine is available as a dietary supplement and is approved by the FDA as a food additive, it is important to note that NO safety studies have been conducted on long-term application to human skin. So there is no information on this at present." (VCF, 2013)

Stem Cells

Stems cells are undifferentiated cells that can become a specialized cell under the right conditions. Most people know of embryonic stem cells, the multipurpose cells that are used as the embryo transforms into an infant. But there are stem cells hidden in adults in what they call "niches". In the skin, at the base of hair follicles, there are niches which are rich in melanocyte stem cells. In vitiligo, these stem cells are thought to be activated by topical treatments such as tacrolimus. Visual support for this is the repigmentation which spreads from hair follicles and first looks like freckles on the treated vitiligo lesions.

Surgical transplants of hair follicles is commonly used for replanting hair on bald spots. Now the same technique is being used for vitiligo. Useful in treating small lesions in areas with hair, individual hair follicles are teased from skin biopsy and implanted using a small needle. The area repigments and the skin color is reported to be an excellent match to the area's normal skin. (Keshavamurthy, 2014)

2. Continuing studies

Studies of the efficacy of existing or potential therapies and combinations of them continue. Some of them are listed below:

- Surgical needling combined with corticosteroids
- Micrografting techniques including one study of minigrafting on the back of the hands comparing two phototherapies.
- Red Light
- UVA1
- Psorolen UVA compared with UVB
- Comparison of topical tacrolimus, pimocrolimus, and local mometasone furoate (Class III corticosteroid)
- A group at the University Hospital Ghent has a model of creating new Koebner's Phenomenon on patients with half or more of their skin depigmented. They use these new areas to test several different treatments on the same patient.
- Comparison of topical tacrolimus, and local mometasone furoate (Class III corticosteroid)
- nbUVB plus PUVA
- nbUVB plus tacrolimus
- Pseudocatalase
- Ginkgo biloba plus nbUVB
- Numerous corticosteroids with or without phototherapy

3. Basic research

There have been two developments in the basic science of vitiligo that keep all of us interested in the disease excited and hopeful.

Gene Therapy

The genetics of vitiligo are not the simple arithmetic of Mendel's peas and human eye color. There appear to be many genes involved as well as environmental factors in and outside the body.

A few basics:

A gene is the basic unit of heredity. Genes, which are made up of DNA, contain instructions to make proteins. Humans have between 20,000 and 25,000 genes.

The genes are located on 23 chromosomes.

A locus (plural loci) is the specific location of a gene, DNA sequence, or position on a chromosome.

The study of the genetic basis of generalized vitiligo has progressed from tracing geographic and family clusters to now finding loci, which are related to vitiligo. The latest studies have been possible through advances in research procedures such that whole genome (all a person's genetic material) of people with vitiligo can be compared with those who do not have the condition, so areas of interest can be pinpointed to study in greater detail. At least 36 loci (those small areas on a chromosome) have been identified which indicate susceptibility for vitiligo. Most of the loci are near genes, which regulate the immune process while about 10% are related to melanocyte chemistry. Many of the loci are also found in patients with other autoimmune diseases.

A large study to identify causal genes is now being carried out by Dr. Richard Spritz at the University of Colorado Health School and VitGene, an international consortium of researchers and vitiligo support organizations in 18 countries. Genetic material from 3,000 people with generalized vitiligo are now being collected in the US and Canada.

And then what? In gene therapy, once the detailed link from a loci to the chemical process that's involved, the holy grail is to be able to locate and replace or destroy a "bad" gene, or add new genetic material to produce a protein to combat a disease. Just knowing the chemical details, however, gives researchers direction for new therapies. Dr. Spritz even dreams of being able to prevent vitiligo through this research. (Spritz,

HSP70iQ435A

I hope they eventually give HSP70iQ435A a better name! First, some background.

Many of the therapies now used for treating vitiligo are "borrowed" from other conditions such as psoriasis. In recent decades, the science of vitiligo has progressed. Its autoimmune nature has been proved through genetic studies. T-cells – which are supposed to protect the body against viruses and bacteria as well as cancerous cells – have been shown to turn against melanocytes and kill them – thereby causing vitiligo patches.

Further research found that HSP70i (heat shock protein 70 – inducible) is activated by stress and triggers the T-cell response in vitiligo. Dr. Caroline LePoole and other scientists at Loyola University first did research into the heat shock proteins and proved that HSP70i was the only one involved in vitiligo. Then they modified the protein by one of its 641 amino acids, from Q435 to Q435A. The team found the same response using cultured human skin. (Mosenson, 2013)

They worked with two mouse vitiligo models. One strain has dark fur but develops white patches when 6-9 months old. When the modified protein was injected into these mice when they were young, none developed white fur patches.

The other mouse strain they use develop the white fur patches soon after birth. They let the mice form these white patches then injected the modified protein. Most of the mice quickly regained their dark fur.

Translating this discovery to a workable human drug is a long process. The lab has applied for US and international patents for the modified protein. Then comes the fund raising for further animal research, regulatory approvals, and human trials.

Chapter 10: Vitiligo Community

The sudden appearance of white spots comes often as a shock to patients and their families. Many are overwhelmed by all the medical terms and decisions they must make. Where to turn for support and information?

1. Vitiligo Support Organizations

Vitiligo support organizations provide understandable medical and research facts. (Full contact information for these organizations is in Appendix C.) Services differ but may include:

- Patient written or video stories
- Physician names who specialize in vitiligo
- Organized groups which meet in several cities
- Access to patient-to-patient chats, some of which are monitored to avoid passing misinformation
- Research funding
- Advocacy
- Pamphlets and newsletters

A few of the websites are described below. These are not-for-profit organizations, which can be relied upon to provide information about both standard and alternative treatments. If anyone is tempted to try a miracle treatment or, through lack of funds, wants to try a do-it-yourself treatment, many of these sites have information about them. It breaks my heart to see discussions on blogs of general sites and the misinformation that is shared there.

NVF – National Vitiligo Foundation, Inc.

NVF efforts include research, education and advocacy. They are setting up chapters in US cities, with 9 chapters underway.

Website features:

- Focused on children and teens; suggests ways to handle the diagnosis
- Good summary of vitiligo and its treatment
- Physician locator. When I visited the site the search system was being repaired.
- There is a sliding fee scale to use the web's information base. At no charge, a person can join an NVFI chapter. $60 gives access to "Ask the Expert" via YouTube.
  Higher fees provide greater access to the organization. Physicians, for $25-$60, have access to the MD-only section of the website and have their contact information made available.
- Offers pamphlets, a handbook for schools and another for patients. The bookstore lists 17 books available on Amazon.

AVRF – American Vitiligo Research Foundation

AVRF focuses on children and families. It supports research and public information efforts.

Website features:

- Story areas of children, teens, and parents experiences.
- Basic facts about vitiligo and treatment
- Progress reports of research AVRF is supporting
- There is no fee for membership

Vitiligo Society UK

Website features:

- Text and video stories of patients
- Mini e-books on 15 topics to read online or download (free)
- Is on Facebook and Twitter
- Section for professionals open to everyone: links to recent research findings; UK issues in patient access to dermatologists; guidelines for general practitioners, and links to journals with vitiligo content.
- There's a membership only section (£26.00/year) with access to more videos and shared content as well as emailed newsletters and a book.

VSI - Vitiligo Support International, USA

VSI is involved in research, information, education, advocacy, and support of individuals.

An online quarterly newsletter covers treatment, reimbursement issues, research results, and open clinical trials. A Q&A section debunks myths and answers specific treatment questions.

Website features:

- Independent support groups in 15 US cities plus London, Sydney, and Toronto
- Moderated forums covering age-specific, general, treatment, alternate treatment, ethnic/language, and gender/dating issues. Non-members can read the discussions; member can participate in them.
- Bookstore offers 14 books for sale.
- Stories by parents, children, and teens
- Detailed information about vitiligo and treatments. Very detailed FAQs.
- Doctor search by US state. Each physician has been nominated by at least one satisfied patient
- Registering on the site provides access to most information on the site with no fee. There is a $25 fee to become a supporting

member with access to an additional chat room, special online forums, special email question contact form and photo gallery.

Skin Conditions Campaign Scotland

This is not a Vitiligo-specific site but the home page notes that only 200 or the 4,960 GPs in Scotland have proper training in dermatology while treating half of all skin conditions. Dermatology is no longer compulsory for trainee GPs.

This made me curious about the US. In the United States, non-dermatologists treat 60% of outpatients with skin, hair, or nail diseases. Federman et al reviewed studies published between 1980-1997 that compared the diagnostic accuracy between dermatologists and other physicians. They reviewed 8 studies that used color slides, transparencies, computer images, or actual patients. Dermatology residents were 91% correct; practicing dermatologists, 96%; family practice residents, 48%; family practice attending physicians, 70%; internal medicine residents, 45%; internal medicine attending physicians, 52%. (Federman, 1997)

2. Suggestions from Patients and Parents

- Learn as much as you can about vitiligo.
- Take care of medical issues such as providing early treatment to stop active vitiligo. Watch for triggers and use sunscreen.
- Visit the different support organizations and join a Facebook group; use these for information about the disease, treatment guidance, help in finding a physician, and making contact with other parents or patients.
- These organizations have booklets to show a child's teacher and adults explaining vitiligo. They have great practical hints on how to role-play with your child if nosy people bother them. (One child on her own printed cards explaining vitiligo and handed them out.)

- Parents – let your child lead. If he or she is not concerned about the patches and you are – don't let them know. Get the facts about vitiligo yourself and provide your child with true explanations in short sentences. There are booklets and sections of the vitiligo support websites, which are especially for children and for teens.
- Vitiligo is not a 'cosmetic' problem. The severity of the disease as judged by a physician may not match with your or your child's perception. If depressed or anxious over the disease, seek help. If you or your child wants to cover the "spots" – get some help from camouflage experts or aestheticians. Children as young as 6 years old have been taught to use camouflage makeup independently.
- Find a good doctor. Don't be put off by one who is clueless. Many patients find a helpful doctor who is perhaps not well versed in vitiligo treatment but who is willing to learn. Through your contacts you can provide help for him or her.

3. Medical literature

I urge patients and families to do research on the disease. Get used to the language. Much of the material is available on the website of vitiligo support organizations such as those described above. Sometimes specific issues can't be covered by these postings. You can use regular search engines like Yahoo and Google, but when I'm trying to find a medical article I generally start with Medscape or Google Scholar.

Medscape

Medscape is a good place to start. The website is free. Searches can be made in 3 categories: News and Perspective, Drugs and Diseases, and CME/Education. Most articles that pop up can be accessed directly while some require registration.

Google Scholar

Google scholar searches can be narrowed to return journal articles for specific years. Many of the articles returned by the search are not attainable or are expensive to see, but others are freely available. Sometimes in the right column of the search results there is a PDF form of the article that's available free.

4. Facebook

I see two large groups on Facebook that are closed to members only. Both have administrators that are available to members. I have not looked at the sites.

Vitiligo Pride: With 2900 members, Vitiligo Pride's motto is "We Love Our Spots"

Vitiligo: With 5600 member, Vitiligo has an international membership and its banner is "It's Just Vitiligo".

5. Books

There are books on vitiligo and books on people's experience with vitiligo. One that may be useful to patients is *My Victory against Vitiligo* by Xichao Mo. Published in 2014, Mo's experience may be typical of many patients: treatments started and stopped; dermatologist's telling him there was no treatments; trials of a homemade remedy. In the end, he was treated successfully with diet management, topical calcineurin inhibitor (Protopic and Elidel), sunlight and nbUVB, and dietary supplements.

6. Celebrities

I was never terribly cute growing up and found solace in seeing the childhood photos of famous people. As vitiligo affects 1% or so of the population, it affects well-known people as well as the rest of us. Michael Jackson may be the most well known of celebrities with vitiligo, but there are many others. Just a few are listed below:

- Graham Norton, a British TV presenter/ comedian

- Lee Thomas, a TV anchorman. He has made several YouTube videos, including his experience in Jordan with Dr. Schallreuter and Scenesse treatment. His book Turning White was published in 2007. Thomas turned completely white then has undergone treatment with Scenesse, which has been fairly effective.
- Bryan Danielson, an American pro wrestler. Vitiligo affects his face, which he covers with tanning cream.
- Jon Hamm, actor. Perhaps best known for his role in Mad Men, the stress of the show brought vitiligo lesions to his hands. This was his first experience with the disease.
- Rasheed Wallace, retired NBA basketball player. Wallace has lesions on his head, hands, and legs.
- Big Krizz Kaliko, a US rapper. Born Samuel William Christopher Watson, Big Krizz Kaliko Vitiligo is his full stage name. He named his debut album "Vitiligo".
- Doc Hammer, co-creator of "Venture Bros". Season 6 of the animated comedic drama is scheduled for 2015.
- John Henson, comedian and TV actor/writer/host/producer. Henson is well known for hosting Talk Soup and is now in his 7th season as co-host of Wipeout – the extreme obstacle game.
- Chantelle Brown-Young, international model. A young woman from Toronto, Brown-Young has vitiligo patches everywhere – and models with them. A 2014 contestant on America's Next Top Model, she was picked on growing up and was determined to beat the bullies. She has a video on YouTube, "Vitiligo: A skin condition, not a life changer".
- Dudley Moore, Composer, Comedian, Musician, Film Producer, Screenwriter. Famous as Arthur and his work on

"Beyond the Fringe", and in several movies including "Arthur". Moore died in 2002.

- Steve Martin, comedian, actor, and banjo player. He had prematurely grey hair, often linked with vitiligo.

- Richard Hammond, British presenter, radio host, writer and journalist. Known for his part TV's "Top Gear" and "Brainiac: Science Abuse."

Chapter 11: Costs & Reimbursement

The cost of vitiligo treatment depends, among other variables, upon the extent of the lesions, whether the disease is just starting or has developed into widespread lesions, whether the first treatments work and stop any active disease and repigment the lesions, or whether the first treatments fail and other treatments are attempted. Where a person lives also has an effect upon costs, cities tending to be more expensive. Cities also have the greater resources and may have more treatments to offer patients.

Most values are in US dollars. British pound equivalents are given when meaningful – they are not provided when services are available in the UK through the health service.

1. Costs

Physician visits and lab fees

The cost of physician visits will vary by region of the country and within regions. They could range from $50-$200 a visit. With insurance, costs range from $5-$30/visit. Lab fees are well reimbursed if medically necessary.

Pharmaceuticals

Estimates of cost of drugs are from GoodRX for pharmacies in Florida. The costs assumed purchaser took advantage of available coupons and/or discounts.

The website www.fpnotebook.com is a good source for estimating topical medication needs by surface area of vitiligo lesions to be treated – with estimates for adults and children. The chapter for this is "topical medication quantity".

The website drugs.com is a good place to check out drug safety issues.

Topical steroids

Three months of a potent medication such as mometasone furoate is given 3 weeks on and one week off or 68 days total. Total cost would depend upon size of vitiligo lesions. A 45-gram tube costs $25 for the generic drug and about $100 for the Elicon brand. The 45 grams is sufficient for a month's application for an adult face & neck or half of an adult's trunk.

Systemic steroids

Depending upon the length of treatment, dexamethasone is given two days a week for 26 weeks would cost $25-$50.

Topical calcineurin inhibitors

The two medications used for vitiligo are pimocrolimus (brand name Elidel) and tacrolimus (brand name Protopic). Both drugs are expensive but fortunately are applied to form a very thin layer on the skin.

Valeant has a manufacturer's assistance program for Elidel – for those with no insurance covering pharmaceuticals and with low incomes, six months of the drug may be available at no cost. Income guidelines are subject to change but are about $39,000 for a family of three.

Costs for 30 gm tubes of each drug: Elidel $204, Protopic, $235. Both cost estimates are with discounts and/or coupons at a US pharmacy.

Neither drug is yet available in generic form. Some formulations may be available online, so please read the notice below about the dangers of buying them:

Notification at Drugs.com: "Fraudulent online pharmacies may attempt to sell an illegal generic version of Protopic. These medications may be counterfeit and potentially unsafe. If you purchase medications online, be sure you are buying from a reputable and valid online pharmacy. Ask your health care provider for advice if you are unsure about the online purchase of any medication."

Depigmentation chemical

Monobenzone ethyl ester in a cream is the most commonly prescribed depigmentation chemical. In the US, Benoquin was the only brand available and was available as an over-the-counter product. The manufacturer, ICN/Valeant, stopped producing Benoquin some years ago. The usual concentration is 20% in a skin cream. Some web sites still are selling old Benoquin stock; and complaints have been made that the expiration dates have gone by. Some overseas companies use Benoquin as if it were the common name for the compound. Other patients have had online drugs tested and they've been contaminated with heavy metals. As it may take several months or more to fully depigment and there are so many complications associated with depigmentation, many physicians refer patients to compounding pharmacies. My advice is to follow the physician's advice on what is available locally that is safe.

Costs will vary.

Office nbUVB treatment

Costs will depend upon the area needing treatment and the length of treatment. Generally, at least three months of twice weekly treatment is given before deciding the treatment isn't effective. If effective, treatment can last as long as two years. Shorter treatments are now being experienced for smaller lesions when topical agents combined with phototherapy.

Phototherapy costs vary from about $20 to $60.

Lowest cost, i.e. treatment stopped because no repigmentation occurred: $520-$1,560.

Treatment successful in 6 months: $1,040 – $3,120.

Treatment successful in 1 year: $2,080 – $6,240

Treatment successful in 2 years: $4,140 – $12,480

Office excimer laser or lamp

Excimer laser treatments are more expensive than nbUVB as a direct result of the higher purchase cost of the equipment. The laser is used on smaller lesions and treatments cost about $100-$200 per treatments. Length of treatment is much less than for nbUVB.

Excimer lamp (often called excimer systems) cost a tenth of the laser to acquire and don't have the high operating costs of the laser. Cost for these treatments should be closer to nbUVB.

Assuming 24 laser treatments given over 12 weeks, cost would be $2,400 – $4,800.

Home nbUVB

Home nbUVB lights are available in many configurations: wands for small lesions; larger panels for hands, feet, and larger lesions; single full-length panels; and wraparound assembly of four full-length panels. Costs for new equipment range from $600 to $8,000 (370-5000£). There are several companies that offer refurbished equipment at lower costs.

Surgery

Highly variable, depending upon technique and size of area, whether anesthesia is used, and how many treatments are needed. $6,500 – $24,000.

2. Reimbursement

Much advance has been made in having US insurance companies pay for vitiligo treatment but payment is still often denied at first with partial payment made only after concerted effort by the physician office staff and patients.

Vitiligo Support International (VSI) surveyed its members in 2013 about their success in receiving reimbursement. As reported in their Spring 2014 newsletter, on the first application for coverage, only 32% had a positive outcome, ranging from 50% of topical steroids approved compared to only 20% approval for laser therapy treatments. After appeal, 100% received at least partial reimbursement for their care. The patient or family have to be active in use of their health insurance – be aware of which services need prior approval, for example. Or what process is involved in getting approval for phototherapy beyond the initial approved treatments. VSI provided sample appeal letters in the Spring 2014 newsletter.

In searching for a dermatologist, often the larger offices are better able to negotiate with insurance companies. They've already fought the battles. Some offices warn patients not to mention the mental trauma of the disease or how they want to improve their looks: this gives the insurance company reason to deny a claim as a cosmetic one.

Even within the same insurance companies there will be variations in their treatment of requests for coverage.

Some common trends in insurance coverage:

119

Topical and systemic corticosteroids, nbUVB, PUVA, and physician visit

These services are most likely to be covered, although many companies will have rules on the length of treatments and the need to try one or another treatment first.

Excimer laser and lamp

The FDA has approved this phototherapy for vitiligo and many insurance companies now cover it. There will be limits on the length of treatment. Some have requirements that other treatments should be tried first such as failing a 2-month trial of topical agents with or without phototherapy.

Home nbUVB

Some insurance companies will not pay for home units, considering them a safety risk. Other plans have accepted home units as less costly and have protocols for physician oversight. And still other plans will allow home therapy units if the patients has to travel extraordinary distances for treatment.

Many of the phototherapy light companies have reimbursement specialists on staff; many also offer time payments for lights.

Experimental

Many of the suggested treatments for vitiligo are considered experimental. Insurance companies quote the Cochrane reports about the shortcomings of research trials. Treatments often considered in this category are:

- Vitamin D analogs (Calcitriol and paricalcitol)
- Tumor necrosis factor – alpha agents (adalimubab, ethanercept, infliximab)
- CD20 (chimeric monoclonal antibody – vituximab)

- Skin grafting
- Melanocyte grafting

Cosmetic

Most insurance companies deem depigmentation a cosmetic treatment and won't cover it. Nor do they cover medical tattooing and other camouflage agents.

FDA approvals

Many of the drugs used for vitiligo have been approved for diseases other than vitiligo. Some insurance companies won't cover these, which includes the very effective calcineurin inhibitors (Protopic and Elidel), which is FDA-approved for eczema. Vitiligo patients form a very small percentage of patients using these drugs, making it not cost effective for pharmaceutical companies to perform the studies required for a broader FDA approval.

Chapter 12: Mental Health and Vitiligo

Psychological stress often triggers the onset of vitiligo; it also may trigger flare-ups. Some patients with vitiligo suffer psychological issues during their lives. It's important for both patients, families, and their physicians to be aware of this and provide help if needed.

1. Psychological stress as trigger

The relation of psychological stress to autoimmune skin diseases has been known for centuries. For instance, the physician to a prince of Persia in 1700 BC diagnosed the prince's psoriasis as stemming from anxiety over succeeding his father. (Shafii, 1979)

Psychological stress had long been assumed to be one of the triggers of vitiligo and most studies have confirmed this. Examples of stressors identified have included death of a family member or close friend; divorce or separation of parents; moving away from relatives, friends, or country; beginning school or changing schools or jobs. Fights and heated arguments have also been mentioned by patients.

2. Mental Health Issues: Living with Vitiligo

Vitiligo can be a life-changing disease. There is an initial first patch, then the worry about spreading or recurrences. And then the need to face the foggy uncertainty of treatments: one study of children's mental health found the 74 kids had received 27 different treatments among them.

Vitiligo brings aggravations. Vitiligo means being careful in the sun. It itches, especially in the beginning of generalized vitiligo. Treatments take time and require patience and money. Not all physicians know how to treat it. Strangers mention it if the patches are visible. Children get bullied. Women in India hide their condition before marriage as it is such a stigma. Patients who want to hide their patches endure more treatments if the first don't work; they dress to avoid revealing patches; they avoid swimming and dressing rooms. If subject to Koebner phenomenon (patches from pressure or friction), some sports such as horse riding and wearing tight clothes are avoided and simple things like using a laptop and resting the wrist on the machine brings more white patches.

There have been many studies to measure the quality of life among different groups of patients. The studies have used existing quality of life questionnaires for dermatology patients (the DLQI – Dermatology Life Quality Index) or a generic ones for any situation. Şenol et al. (2013) have been developing a vitiligo-specific index, Vitiligo Life Quality Index or VLQI. (Şenol, 2013)

Why is it important to measure the quality of life? For one thing, the patient's perception of the severity of the disease may differ from the physician's. In studies of adults and adolescents, the patients' quality of life is more a factor of their fears about vitiligo and their personality than the severity of vitiligo itself. With quality of life measures, which can be a simple perceived severity scale, the physician can stay alert and refer for counseling or other mental health services if needed. In addition, Parsad (2003) found that patients with higher DLQI scores had less favorable treatment outcomes and suggested that "Improving the physician's interpersonal skills with the vitiligo patients increases patient's satisfaction and consequently may have a positive effect on adherence to treatment protocol and better outcome of treatments".

For another reason, quality-of-life scores are important for determining the effects of treatment, both for research purposes and for clinical practice.

The DLQI is a self-administered form of ten questions about vitiligo's effect upon the patient during the prior week. The scale runs from 0-3 with 0 being no effect and 3 being very much affected. The overall score runs from zero to 30. There is a modified instrument (CDLQI) for children, which is given in either text or cartoon form. A vitiligo-specific index is also being developed.

3. Comparison of Vitiligo DLQI with other skin conditions

In a summary of ten years' experience of DLQI, Lewis and Finlay (2004) summarized DLQI results by disease. Data is given as a range of each study's average and then an average of the averages. Later studies show similar relationships, with vitiligo patients as a whole being less affected than some with the other skin conditions.

Condition	No. Studies	No. Patients	Range of Averages	Ave. of Averages
Atopic eczema	12	1409	4.5 – 21.4	12.2
Acne	3	836	4.3 – 17.7	11.9
Psoriasis	11	2460	1.7 – 18.2	8.8
Vitiligo	3	856	4.8 – 15.0	5.6

4. Studies of Camouflage

Ongenae et al (2005) studied 62 vitiligo patients before and one month after camouflage instruction. The DLQI was 7.3 ± 5.6 before and 5.9 ± 5.2 after camouflage. Regardless of overall total depigmented area, patients with face, head and neck involvement had higher scores.

Tanioka et al (2010) also studied vitiligo patients before and one month after camouflage instruction. This study also included control vitiligo patients. The DLQI of the controls increased (concerns about their condition increased) for the controls, going from 3.18 to 4.36. The DLQI of patients receiving camouflage instruction and performing camouflage decreased from 5.90 to 4.48.

5. Children and Teenagers

Krüger et al (2014) studied the effects of vitiligo on the mental health of children and teenagers from Germany and the US using the Children's Dermatology Life Quality Index (CDLQI). The patients were mostly fair skinned: on the Fitzpatrick scale, 82% had types I-III and 17.6% had types IV-V. None had skin type VI. There were 54 children and 18 teenagers. The CDLQI did not differ by age.

The average CDLQI score was low, 2.8, but higher than the controls' 0.6. The lower scores are explained by the group's fairly pale skin. But subsets of the group scored higher, especially those with extensive involvement of the face (average score 5.5) and those who reported being picked on or receiving nasty comments (average score 10.5). Those who had family members with vitiligo (35% of the total) scored lower (were less affected) than those who did not.

6. Comparison of Vitiligo Quality of life/Depression/Anxiety with two other conditions

In a study in Egypt, Saleh et al. studied 150 patients in three groups of 50: vitiligo, psoriasis, and alopecia areata (AA). In addition to the DQLI questionnaire they used other standard tests of anxiety and depression. (Saleh, 2008}

The average DLQI and the range of values for the three conditions is shown below:

Patient Group	DLQI Range	DLQI Average
Vitiligo	3-21	10.9
Psoriasis	4-27	13.7
AA	2-20	9.1

The mental health data collected are shown below for the three conditions. The psychiatric morbidity numbers are in range for studies of vitiligo patients is Western Europe; higher numbers have been reported for India (55% - 75%).

Mental Health Issue	Vitiligo	Psoriasis	AA
Psychiatric morbidity	34%	35%	36%
Anxiety	14%	12%	24%
Depression	24%	30%	16%
Suicide threats	6%	8%	6%
Suicide attempts	2%	4%	2%

The total body surface area covered by vitiligo patches ranged from 4 – 50%, averaging 19% ± 11. As part of the assessment, the authors collected data on those who had threatened suicide. This group had much greater than average skin involvement: 29% ± 14.

7. Help for patients and family

Experts in the field recognize the psychological burden on many with vitiligo. Guidelines for care developed by the European Dermatology Forum Consensus (2013 for example), state: "For *all* subtypes of disease or lines of treatment, psychological support and counseling, including access to camouflage instructors, is needed."

But no specific mental health approach has been recommended. There have been two small, randomly controlled trials of cognitive behavioral therapy (CBT). Papadopoulos (1999) studied the effect of one-to-one CBT in adults, 8 in the treatment group and 8 controls. The treatment group received a 1-hour session a week for 8 weeks. The control group had no treatment. Follow-ups for 5 months showed improvement in the quality of life, self-esteem and body image. (In fact their scores were normal.) The patients not receiving any medical treatment for vitiligo also had photographs of their vitiligo and the area involved were sized by computer. Those in the CBT group each experienced a reduction of vitiligo area from 26%-35% while two in the untreated group experience an increase in vitiligo area.

In a later study, Papadopoulos (2004) found that group CBT and group patient-centered therapy for vitiligo patients did not work under the conditions of the study.

What is CBT? This is a short-term treatment with a therapist to deal with a specific problem. Therapists and patients challenge the patient's beliefs and develop coping strategies. Therapy doesn't include drugs but does include relaxation techniques. It differs from patient-centered therapy in that the therapist directly challenges the patient's beliefs.

8. What do patients say?

When questioning adults whose vitiligo started as children, they wished they had had more information about vitiligo in the beginning and contact with others with the condition as they were growing up.

Now with the Internet, there is almost too much information available! There are support groups in many cities and virtual online support groups wherever there's an Internet connection. If there isn't an Internet connection at home, neighbors, libraries, and schools have them.

A survey of members of the UK Vitiligo Society found that only 12.5% of patients got their vitiligo information from dermatologist. The others relied upon the Society or the Internet.

Going through one or several of the major vitiligo support organizations is the safer way to get information and to make contacts with others with vitiligo. These organizations can help locate physicians who treat vitiligo patients. They provide warnings about scams. Most can be contacted directly with questions and concerns. Most of their websites provide opportunities for children, teens, and adults to chat on various topics and trade experiences. These websites and some Facebook groups are monitored to assure misinformation isn't shared.

Through these organizations, young kids and teens now have "pen pals" or Skype with other children all over the world.

Appendices and References

Appendix A

Chemicals Associated with Chemical Leukoderma

Most potent phenol/catechol derivatives
Monobenzyl ether of hydroquinone

Hydroquinone (1,4-dihydroxybenzene; 1,4-benzenediol; quinol; *p*-hydroxyphenol)

p-tert-Butylchatechol

p-tert-Butylphenol

p-tert-Amylphenol

Additional phenol/catechol derivatives
Monomethyl ether of hydroquinone (*p*-methoxyphenol; *p*-hydroxyanisole)

Monoethyl ether of hydroquinone (*p*-ethoxyphenol)

p-Phenylphenol

p-Octylphenol

p-Nonylphenol

p-Isopropylcatechol

p-Methylcatechol

Butylated hydroxytoluene

Butylated hydroxyanisole

Pyrocatechol (1,2-benxenediol)

p-Cresol

Sulfhydryls
β-Mercaptoethylamine hydrochloride (cysteamine)

N-(2-mercaptoethyl)-dimethylamine hydrochloride

Sulfanolic acid

Cystamine dihydrochloride

3-Mercaptopropylamine hydrochloride

Miscellaneous

Mercurials

Arsenic

Cinnamic aldehyde

p-Pheylenediamine

Benzyl alcohol

Azaleic acid

Soymilk and derived protein Thiotepa (inhibits PAR-2)

Brilliant lake red
Fluorouracil Azaleic acid
Tretinoin

Ammoniated mercury

Benzoyl peroxide

Eserine (physostigmine)

Diisopropyl fluorophoshate

Tio-tepa (N, N′, N″-triethylene-thiophosphoramide)

Guanonitrofuracin

Systemic medications

Chloroquine

Fluphenazine (prolixin)

Adapted from:

Raymond E. Boissy and Prashiela Manga. (2004) *On the Etiology of Contact/Occupational Vitiligo* Pigment Cell Research Volume 17, Issue 3, pages 208–214.

Appendix B

Estimates of percentage of skin surface area by major body component.

Treatment options often differ by area of skin affected and the age of patients. For reference, the table below provides an estimate of skin surface area by major body part.

Adult

	Surface area		Surface area
Anterior head	4.5%	Posterior head	4.5%
Anterior torso	18.0%	Posterior torso	18.0%
Anterior leg, each	9.0%	Posterior leg, each	9.0%
Anterior arm, each	4.5%	Posterior arm, each	4.5%
Genitalia/perineum	1.0%		

Child

	Surface area		Surface area
		Anterior head	9%
Posterior head	9%	Anterior torso	18%
Posterior torso	18%	Anterior leg, each	6.75%
Posterior leg, each	6.75%	Anterior arm, each	4.5%
Posterior arm, each	4.5%	Genitalia/perineum	1%

Adult, over 80 kg (177 lb.)

	Surface area		Surface area
Head and neck	2%	Anterior torso	25%
Posterior torso	25%	Leg, each	20%
Arm, each	5%	Genitalia/perineum	0%

Infant weighing less than 10 kg (22 lb)

	Surface area		Surface area
Head and neck	20%	Anterior torso	16%
Posterior torso	16%	Leg, each	16%
Arm, each	8%	Genitalia/perineum	1%

References

O'Sullivan, Susan B., Schmitz, Thomas J. Physical Rehabilitation. 5th ed. F.A. Davis Company, Philadelphia, 2007. p. 1098, Fig 27.9.

Wikipedia

Appendix C

Vitiligo Support Organizations

NVF – National Vitiligo Foundation, Inc.

www.mynvfi.org

AVRF – American Vitiligo Research Foundation

Vitiligo@avrf.org

Vitiligo Society UK

www.vitiligosociety.org.uk

VSI - Vitiligo Support International, USA

www.vitiligosupport.org

VR Foundation

www.vrfoundation.org

Skin Conditions Campaign Scotland

E-mail: info@skinconditionscampaignscotland.org

Changing Faces

www.changingfaces.org.uk

SKIN CAMOUFLAGE SERVICE

Email skincam@changingfaces.org.uk.

British Association of Skin Camouflage

www.vitiligobond.org

Appendix D

Diseases considered autoimmune or autoimmune-related by the American Autoimmune Related Diseases Association

Autoimmune and Autoimmune-Related Diseases

Acute Disseminated Encephalomyelitis (ADEM)

Acute necrotizing hemorrhagic leukoencephalitis

Addison's disease

Agammaglobulinemia

Alopecia areata

Amyloidosis

Ankylosing spondylitis

Anti-GBM/Anti-TBM nephritis

Antiphospholipid syndrome (APS)

Autoimmune angioedema

Autoimmune aplastic anemia

Autoimmune dysautonomia

Autoimmune hepatitis

Autoimmune hyperlipidemia

Autoimmune immunodeficiency

Autoimmune inner ear disease (AIED)

Autoimmune myocarditis

Autoimmune oophoritis

Autoimmune pancreatitis

Autoimmune retinopathy

Autoimmune thrombocytopenic purpura (ATP)

Autoimmune thyroid disease

Autoimmune urticaria

Axonal & neuronal neuropathies

Balo disease

Behcet's disease

Bullous pemphigoid

Cardiomyopathy

Castleman disease

Celiac disease

Chagas disease

Chronic fatigue syndrome**

Chronic inflammatory demyelinating polyneuropathy (CIDP)

Chronic recurrent multifocal ostomyelitis (CRMO)

Churg-Strauss syndrome

Cicatricial pemphigoid/benign mucosal pemphigoid

Crohn's disease

Cogans syndrome

Cold agglutinin disease

Congenital heart block

Coxsackie myocarditis

CREST disease

Essential mixed cryoglobulinemia

Demyelinating neuropathies

Dermatitis herpetiformis

Dermatomyositis

Devic's disease (neuromyelitis optica)

Discoid lupus

Dressler's syndrome

Endometriosis

Eosinophilic esophagitis

Eosinophilic fasciitis

Erythema nodosum

Experimental allergic encephalomyelitis

Evans syndrome

Fibromyalgia**

Fibrosing alveolitis

Giant cell arteritis (temporal arteritis)

Giant cell myocarditis

Glomerulonephritis

Goodpasture's syndrome

Granulomatosis with Polyangiitis (GPA) (formerly called Wegener's Granulomatosis)

Graves' disease

Guillain-Barre syndrome

Hashimoto's encephalitis

Hashimoto's thyroiditis

Hemolytic anemia

Henoch-Schonlein purpura

Herpes gestationis

Hypogammaglobulinemia

Idiopathic thrombocytopenic purpura (ITP)

IgA nephropathy

IgG4-related sclerosing disease

Immunoregulatory lipoproteins

Inclusion body myositis

Interstitial cystitis

Juvenile arthritis

Juvenile diabetes (Type 1 diabetes)

Juvenile myositis

Kawasaki syndrome

Lambert-Eaton syndrome

Leukocytoclastic vasculitis

Lichen planus

Lichen sclerosus

Ligneous conjunctivitis

Linear IgA disease (LAD)

Lupus (SLE)

Lyme disease, chronic

Meniere's disease

Microscopic polyangiitis

Mixed connective tissue disease (MCTD)

Mooren's ulcer

Mucha-Habermann disease

Multiple sclerosis

Myasthenia gravis

Myositis

Narcolepsy

Neuromyelitis optica (Devic's)

Neutropenia

Ocular cicatricial pemphigoid

Optic neuritis

Palindromic rheumatism

PANDAS (Pediatric Autoimmune Neuropsychiatric Disorders Associated with Streptococcus)

Paraneoplastic cerebellar degeneration

Paroxysmal nocturnal hemoglobinuria (PNH)

Parry Romberg syndrome

Parsonnage-Turner syndrome

Pars planitis (peripheral uveitis)

Pemphigus

Peripheral neuropathy

Perivenous encephalomyelitis

Pernicious anemia

POEMS syndrome

Polyarteritis nodosa

Type I, II, & III autoimmune polyglandular syndromes

Polymyalgia rheumatica

Polymyositis

Postmyocardial infarction syndrome

Postpericardiotomy syndrome

Progesterone dermatitis

Primary biliary cirrhosis

Primary sclerosing cholangitis

Psoriasis

Psoriatic arthritis

Idiopathic pulmonary fibrosis

Pyoderma gangrenosum

Pure red cell aplasia

Raynauds phenomenon

Reactive Arthritis

Reflex sympathetic dystrophy

Reiter's syndrome

Relapsing polychondritis

Restless legs syndrome

Retroperitoneal fibrosis

Rheumatic fever

Rheumatoid arthritis

Sarcoidosis

Schmidt syndrome

Scleritis

Scleroderma

Sjogren's syndrome

Sperm & testicular autoimmunity

Stiff person syndrome

Subacute bacterial endocarditis (SBE)

Susac's syndrome

Sympathetic ophthalmia

Takayasu's arteritis

Temporal arteritis/Giant cell arteritis

Thrombocytopenic purpura (TTP)

Tolosa-Hunt syndrome

Transverse myelitis

Type 1 diabetes

Ulcerative colitis

Undifferentiated connective tissue disease (UCTD)

Uveitis

Vasculitis

Vesiculobullous dermatosis

Vitiligo

Wegener's granulomatosis (now termed Granulomatosis with Polyangiitis (GPA)

**NOTE: Fibromyalgia and Chronic Fatigue are listed, not because they are autoimmune, but because many persons who suffer from them have associated autoimmune disease(s)

American Autoimmune Related Diseases Association

22100 Gratiot Avenue

Eastpointe, MI 48021-2227

www.aarda.org

References

Alikhan*A. (2010). In *Vitiligo: A comprehensive overview.* Berwyn and Chicago, Illinois; and New York, New York.

Aljasser, M. (n.d.). *Efficacy and Safety of Intralesional Corticosteroids in the Treatment of Vitiligo* . U.S. National Institutes of Health.

Eleftheriadou*, V. (2011). Future research into the treatment of vitiligo: where should our priorities lie? Results of the vitiligo priority setting partnership . *British Journal of Dermatology*, 530–536 .

Esfandiarpour*, I. C.-o. (2012). Dermatologica Sinica . *Dermatologica Sinica* , 43-46.

Federman*, D. (1997). The abilities of primary care physicians in dermatology: implications for quality of care. . *Am J Manag Care*, 1487-92.

Friends, V. C. (Nov 14, 2013). *Vitiligo Cover Friends, Interview with Dr. Soumyanath* . Vitiligo Cover Friends.

Gonzalez*, U. (2011). Guidelines for Designing and Reporting Clinical Trials in Vitiligo . *Arch Dermatol.* , 1428-36.

Goren*, A. (2014). Novel topical cream delivers safe and effective sunlight therapy for vitiligo by selectively filtering damaging ultraviolet radiation . *Dermatologic Therapy*, 195–197 .

Grimes*, P. (2013). The efficacy of afamelanotide and narrowband UV-B phototherapy for repigmentation of vitiligo. . *JAMA Dermatol.* , 68-73.

Harris, J. (2012). *Clinical Trial of Simvastatin to Treat Generalized Vitiligo* . U.S. National Institutes of Health.

Korobko*, I. (2014). Acridone acetic acid, sodium salt, as an agent to stop vitiligo progression: a pilot study. *Dermatologic Therapy* , 219–222.

Krüger*, J. (2014). Disease-related behavioral patterns and experiences affect quality of life in children and adolescents with vitiligo. *International Journal of Dermatology* , 43–50.

Kutlubay*, Z. (2012). Vitiligo as an Autoimmune Disease . *J Turk Acad Dermatol* , 1262-1265.

Lewis*, V. J. (2004). 10 Years Experience of the Dermatology Life Quality Index (DLQI) . *Journal of Investigative Dermatology Symposium Proceedings* , 169–180.

Majid, I. (2010). Topical placental extract: does it increase the efficacy of narrowband UVB therapy in vitiligo? *Indian J Dermatol Venereol Leprol*, 254-258.

Mo, X. (2014). *My Victory Against Vitiligo.* Paclinx Publishing.

Montes*, L. (1992). Folic acid and vitamin B12 in vitiligo: a nutritional approach. *Cutis*, 39-42.

Mosenson*, J. (2013). A central role for inducible heat-shock protein 70 in autoimmune vitiligo. *Experimental Dermatology* , 566–569.

Mulekarl*, S. (2013). Surgical interventions for vitiligo: an evidence-based review . *British Journal of Dermatology, Special Issue: Ethnic Skin* , 57-66.

Ongenae*, K. (2005). Effect of vitiligo on self-reported health-related quality of life . *Br J Dermatol.* , 1165- 1172.

Papadopoulos*, L. (1999). Coping with the disfiguring effects of vitiligo: a preliminary investigation into the effects of cognitive-behavioural therapy. *Br J Med Psychol.* , 385-396.

Papadopoulos*, L. (2004). Living with Vitiligo: A Controlled Investigation into the Effects of Group Cognitive-

Behavioural and Person-Centred Therapies . *Dermatology and Psychosomatics* , 172-177.

Parsad*, D. (2003). Quality of life in patients with vitiligo . *Health Qual Life Outcomes*, 58-60.

Schallreuter*, K. (1991). Low catalase level in the epidermis of patients with vitiligo. *J Invest Dermatol*, 1081-1085.

Shafii*, M. (1979). Exploratory psychotherapy in the treatment of psoriasis. Twelve hundred years ago . *Archives of general psychiatry*, 1242-1245.

Tag*S. (2014). Beyond vitiligo guidelines: combined stratified/personalized approaches for the vitiligo patient . *Experimental Dermatology* , 219-223.

Taieb*, A. (2013). Guidelines for the management of vitiligo: the European Dermatology Forum consensus . *British Association of Dermatologists* , 5–19.

Tanioka*, M. (2010). Camouflage for patients with vitiligo vulgaris improved their quality of life . *Journal of Cosmetic Dermatology* , 72–75.

University, O. H. (2013, 2014). *Black Pepper, Piperine and Vitiligo and Piperine for the Treatment of Vitiligo* . OHSU www.ohsu.edu.

(Nov 14th 2013). *VCF – Vitiligo Cover Friends, Interview with Dr. Soumyanath Nov 14th, 2013.* VCF Vitiligo Cover Friends .

Vinay*, K. (2014). Stem cells in vitiligo: Current position and prospects . *Pigment International*, 8-12.

Yahgoobi*, R. (2011). Vitiligo: a review of the published work. *Journal of Dermatology*, 419-431.

Yoon*J. (2011). Complementary and Alternative Medicine for Vitiligo. In D. K. (Ed.), *Vitiligo - Management and Therapy* (pp. 143-162). http://www.intechopen.com/books.

*Multiple authors not shown

Published by IMB Publishing 2014

Made in the USA
Middletown, DE
23 July 2016